MACRO COOKBOOK FOR MEN

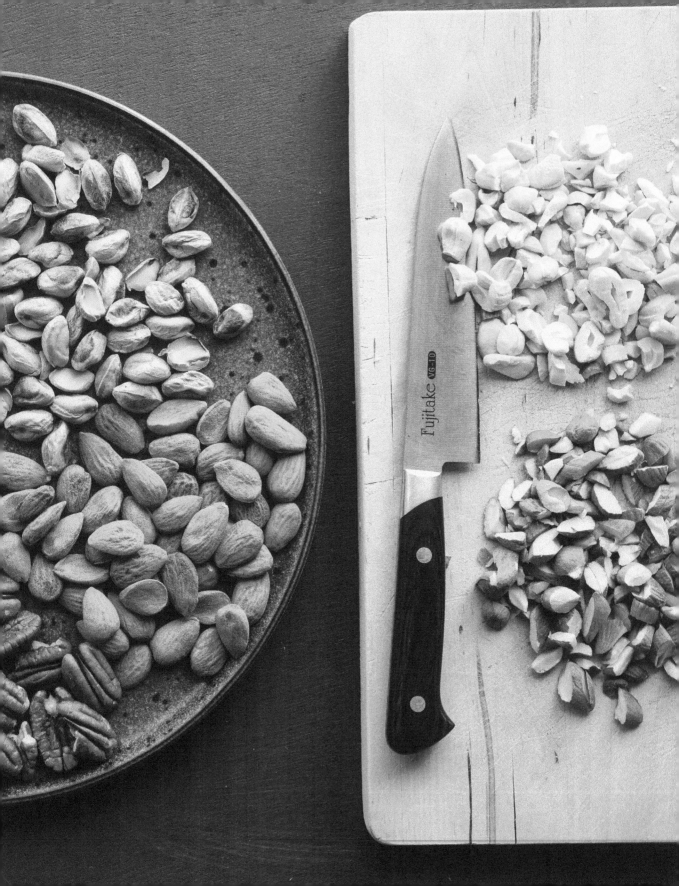

MACRO COOKBOOK FOR MEN

7-Day Meal Plans, Recipes, and Workouts for
Fat Loss and Muscle Gain

Andy De Santis, RD, MPH

ROCKRIDGE
PRESS

This book is dedicated to my dearly departed friend and fitness enthusiast Josh, who would have celebrated his 32nd birthday at the time of my writing this.

Interior and Cover Designer: Jill Lee
Art Producer: Megan Baggott
Editor: Marjorie DeWitt
Production Manager: Riley Hoffman

Cover photo © Klaus Arras/Gräfe & Unzer Verlag/StockFood USA; Marija Vidal, ii, vi, viii, 17, 18, 52, 78; Darren Muir, 34, 36, 38, 56, 58, 72, 76, 80, 102, 104, 106; Thomas J. Story, 54; Johnny Autry, 74

Illustrations, James Pop

Paperback ISBN: 978-1-63807-655-1
eBook ISBN: 978-1-63807-894-4
R0

CONTENTS

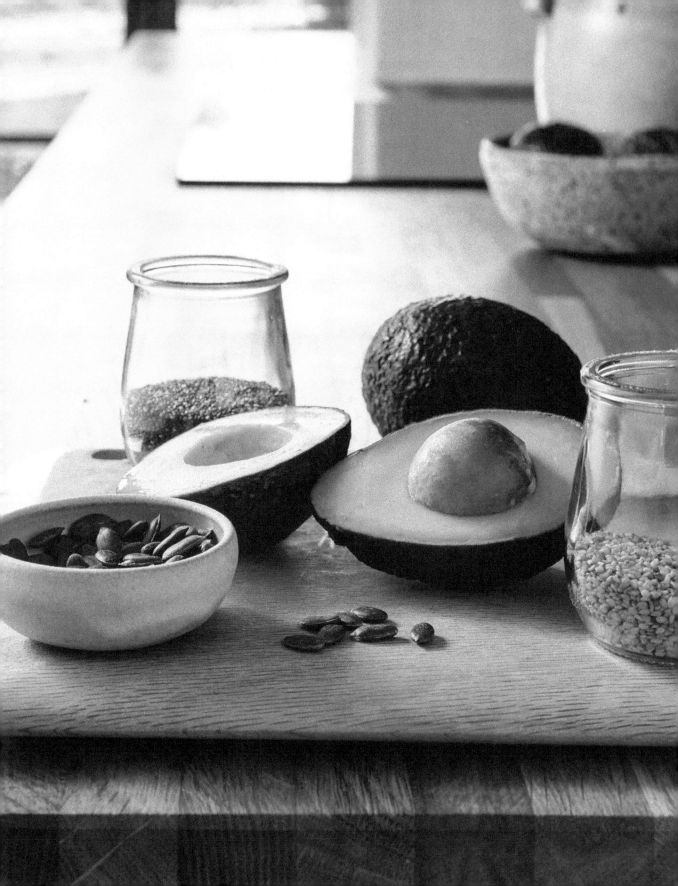

INTRODUCTION

First and foremost, I want to welcome you to the *Macro Cookbook for Men*. My name is Andy De Santis, and I'm a registered dietitian from Toronto with a master's degree in public health nutrition.

This book is my 10th print publication, and I am thrilled to be the one to lead you toward a better understanding of a flexible, yet focused, macronutrient-based approach to eating while also working toward your nutrition and fitness goals. In my five years as a dietician in private practice, I've helped hundreds of men of various fitness backgrounds use a macro-based approach, and I'm very much looking forward to helping you do the same.

Between my teens and 30s, I used better nutrition and fitness practices to significantly improve my strength and overall health, so I approach this book as both the expert with the theoretical and scientific background and perspective and as someone who has been where you are today.

I appreciate your desire to combine a scientific, results-driven approach with the need for a practical and sustainable fitness and nutrition routine. It's important to have flexibility and simplicity when optimizing macronutrient targets. Many of my clients have personal goals focused on altering body composition through muscle gain, fat loss, or both. They rely on me to pave the way to these goals in the most painless manner possible.

That's where the *Macro Cookbook for Men* comes in!

In this book, I will show you how to determine the right macronutrient distribution based on your goals and starting point while also teaching you the key foods and micro-nutrients to use in order to get the most out of your approach. I also offer information on supplements, including the role I think they should play in your routine. This should help you better determine whether they are worth your time.

All of this guidance is supported with 7-day meal plans, exercise plans, and a library of recipes that can be swapped in and out as desired.

Get excited about this journey! Having clear direction with your nutrition goals will provide peace of mind and the confidence to push forward. With a little focus and planning, meaningful progress toward your goals is within reach.

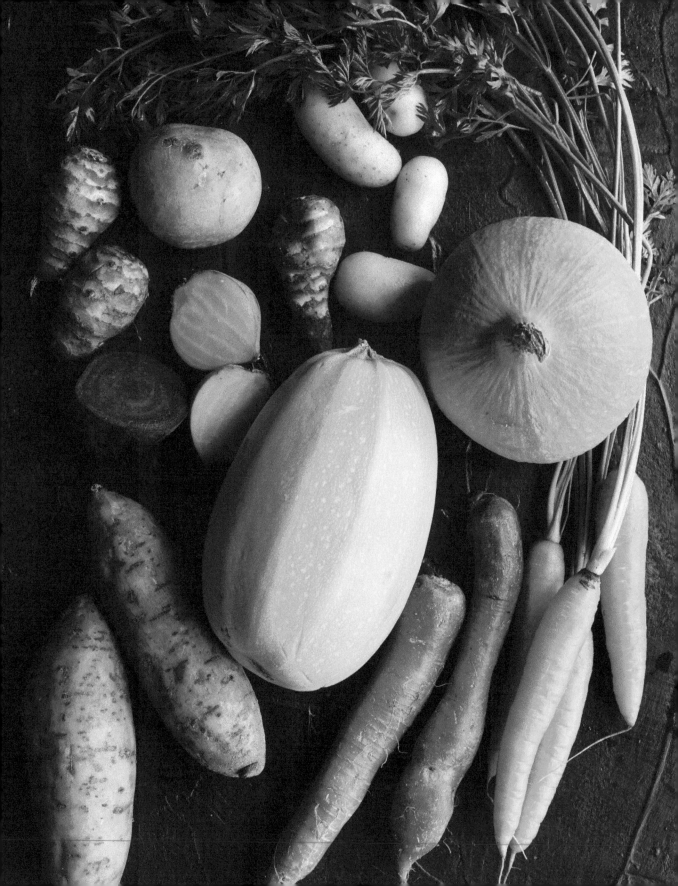

CHAPTER 1

MAKING MACRO WORK FOR YOU

This chapter defines what a macro approach to nutrition entails. It provides a deep dive, supported with scientific data, on how best to craft a strategy that can bring a macro approach to your life in an achievable and sustainable way.

Why Eat This Way?

Having spent a great deal of time advising clients who are new to nutrition and fitness, I appreciate how challenging it can be to make sense of all the wildly different diet guidance that is dispensed online and in social circles. Everyone is a nutrition expert!

General online content seems to favor fitness plans that require the exclusion of the vast majority of favorite foods. Because of this misinformation, clients rely on me to quiet the "nutrition noise" and provide a reliable plan. With this book, we are using a flexible, macro-based approach that will allow for broader caloric and nutrient goals through a wide variety of foods. Sometimes referred to as IIFYM (if it fits your macros), this nutritional approach is appealing because it does not, by definition, exclude any specific foods. Instead, this approach focuses on a scientific framework for estimating energy and nutrient needs relative to fitness goals.

Understanding Fat Loss and Muscle Gain

Generally, a macro-based approach to nutrition appeals to those with body composition goals focused on increasing muscle mass, decreasing body fat, or both. In order to make the most of this approach, it's important to consider macronutrients as well as calories, micronutrients, and meal timing.

How Much You Eat (Calories)

For our purposes, we will discuss calories as food energy that is released during digestion and used by our bodies to meet physiological functions. This includes cellular-level functions and large movements like walking, running, jumping, and all of that good stuff.

Individual calorie needs vary based on a wide number of factors, including: age, gender, height, weight, activity level, and personal fitness goals. For example, a shorter, less active man with a weight-loss goal will have lower caloric requirements than a taller, more active man with a muscle-building goal.

Keep in mind that although caloric content remains relevant, there is much more to food than just calories. I'll explain this more as we move forward in the chapter.

How You Fuel Your Body (Macronutrients)

Most calories that we consume come from one of three macronutrients: carbohydrates, fat, and protein. Carbohydrates are the primary fuel source for the human body and tend to be found in whole foods that are also high in dietary fiber, such as whole grains, starchy vegetables, fruits, and legumes.

Other carbohydrate food items, like baked goods, buns, chips, and pretzels, contain carbohydrates but do not contain much fiber. Carbohydrates are used by the human body regularly during physical activity, and as a result, active people and athletes tend to have higher carbohydrate requirements.

Fats are an alternative fuel source and are required for our bodies to produce important hormones. According to Joseph Whittaker and Kexin Wu in their article about low-fat diets and testosterone in men, those who pursue low-fat diets may suffer decreases in testosterone levels, which could have implications for physical performance and muscle-building capabilities.

Some fat-containing foods, such as nuts, seeds, and avocado, also provide large amounts of fiber and essential minerals. Fish is a great source of a unique and healthy fat known as omega-3s. Fat may also be found in a wide array of other foods, including oils, baked goods, fried foods, and certain types of meat and dairy. The fats from these products have a place in our diet, but they don't carry the same positive health impacts as nuts, seeds, avocado, and fish.

Protein is most famous for its role in building and maintaining muscle, which is why resistance training has higher protein needs than a sedentary lifestyle. Protein is found in various types of meat, eggs, dairy, fish, nuts, seeds, and legumes.

Macronutrients are more than just their caloric value and basic functionality. Protein and fiber, for example, are also important because they aid in satiety, and protein requires more energy to break down than either carbohydrates or fat.

What You Eat (Diet)

A major benefit of a macro-based diet is that there aren't any specific food or food group restrictions. There are, of course, key foods and nutrients that should play a bigger role than others, but there is a lot of freedom of choice in how to best hit caloric and macronutrient goals.

For many people, this is the 80/20 approach to eating, which will be discussed later in the chapter. At this point, it's important to understand that the 80/20 approach simply means 80 percent of a diet should be focused on whole foods, including the recipes provided in chapters 3 through 6. This will aid in getting the micronutrients and antioxidants needed for optimal health while staying satiated and ensuring fiber needs are met, which keeps digestive health on track.

When You Eat (Timing)

Meal timing has become an increasingly hot topic with the rise in popularity of intermittent fasting and the variety of ways to organize the day around food. What matters most is what is eaten, how much is eaten, and the practical aspects of planning and managing meals.

A 2018 study by Brad Schoenfeld shows that the body makes the best use of protein intake when it is spread throughout the day across three or four meals and snacks. It seems that for most people, this approach to eating is generally the easiest and most practical to pull off. Ultimately, meal timing is a personal preference, but it's acceptable if timing looks different on different days.

Determining Your Macros and Calories

The best way to establish the right calorie and macronutrient targets is to start with protein because of its ability to build and maintain muscle mass. The following recommendations come from many respected organizations, such as the National Academy of Sports Medicine, the International Society of Sports Nutrition, and the American College of Sports Medicine.

The optimal range of protein per day for muscle building is between 1.6 and 2 grams per kilogram of body weight per day. This is equivalent to 0.7 to 0.9 grams of protein per pound of body weight. Some people may prefer to have closer to 1 gram of protein per pound of body weight because they enjoy the satiating effect of protein-rich foods or have a preference for more protein in their routine.

Using an average of 0.8 grams of protein per pound of body weight, applied to a 200-pound man, the protein target would be 160 grams per day, or 25 percent of the total caloric intake in a day. We should then target 50 percent of the remaining calories to come from carbohydrates and 25 percent from fat. As long as the protein intake remains at 25 percent and the calorie target is met, it's okay for carbohydrates and fat to fluctuate. Those who enjoy protein-rich foods may boost the protein closer to 35 percent and reduce carbohydrates, but it's not advised to drop any macronutrient below 20 percent, assuming a balanced and diverse diet is desired.

With the macronutrient targets addressed, how do we determine a starting calorie number? That depends on the goals and the starting point. Using the following three cases

THE ROLE OF SUPPLEMENTS

As a dietitian, I prefer to solve nutritional deficiencies through food alone, but when necessary, I won't hesitate to recommend supplementation. The macronutrient targets laid out in this book can be reached primarily using whole foods, although the protein intake suggestions may be a bit higher than customary, or there may be a role for products like protein powders.

From the micronutrient perspective, vitamin D and omega-3 acids are noteworthy, because they are essential nutrients found naturally in very few foods. Those who don't consume fish multiple times a week may struggle to get enough of both. For this reason, this ends up being the supplement combination I recommend most often to my clients. Generally, most other vitamin and mineral inadequacies can be solved using the diet patterns outlined later in this chapter and brought to life via the meal plans in chapter 2.

From a pure fitness and strength perspective, the unfortunate reality is that many supplements aren't scientifically proven to be useful and can come with a hefty price tag. The efficacy of popular products like BCAAs and "testosterone" boosters is not well supported by evidence, but creatine monohydrate, one of the most studied and scientifically supported athletic supplements, is certainly the major exception. As outlined in a 2017 review published in the *Journal of the International Society of Sports Nutrition*, creatine allows muscles to better use energy in short, intense movements like weight-lifting and HIIT (high-intensity interval training) workouts. Over time, this contributes to strength, muscle, and performance gains. Although it can lead to water retention in the short term, this usually resolves itself after a week. The review further suggests that creatine monohydrate be used as follows: consuming 3 grams per kilogram of body weight per day for the first week before consuming 3 to 5 grams daily thereafter.

with men of different goals and starting points, we will start by calculating the basal metabolic rate (BMR) for each.

CASE #1: a man whose goal is to lose body fat

CASE #2: a man whose goal is to add muscle mass

CASE #3: a man whose goal is not clear on which is more pressing

1. Work out Your Basal Metabolic Rate (BMR)

The basal metabolic rate represents the amount of energy expended at rest and is calculated based on height, weight, and age. The formula is listed here, but there is always the option of completing the calculation using an online calculator, such as the one at Active.com/fitness /calculators/bmr.

> **BMR Formula for Men = 88.362 + (13.397 x weight in kg) + (4.799 x height in cm) – (5.677 x age in years)**

In calculating the BMR for each of the aforementioned cases, using a man that is 40 years old and standing 5 feet, 9 inches, we find:

CASE #1: weight 200 lbs., BMR=1,920

CASE #2: weight 130 lbs., BMR=1,495

CASE #3: weight 165 lbs., BMR=1,700

2. Determine Your Activity Level

Activity level impacts how many calories are needed. The higher the activity level, the greater the need for more calories. Using the following multipliers and BMR, the daily caloric need can be calculated as:

Moderate exercise (defined as 3 to 5 days of exercise a week) = BMR x 1.55 = daily calories needed

Very active (6 to 7 days of exercise a week) = BMR x 1.725 = daily calories needed

Extra active (exercise every day of the week combined with a very physical job) = BMR x 1.9 = daily calories needed

Using a moderate activity level (1.55) and varying BMRs sample scenario calculations are:

CASE #1: 1,920 x 1.55 = 2,976 daily calories

CASE #2: 1,495 x 1.55 = 2,317 daily calories

CASE #3: 1,700 x 1.55 = 2,635 daily calories

For each of these scenarios, we would have the following strategies:

CASE #1: For the individual wanting to lose body fat, the caloric target will be reduced to 2,350.

CASE #2: For the individual wanting to gain muscle, the caloric target will be increased to 2,817.

CASE #3: For the individual for whom neither is prioritized above the other, the caloric target will be maintained at 2,635. Some individuals starting at a higher body weight and pursuing muscle gain and fat loss simultaneously may also opt to decrease by an additional 250 calories (keeping the total number closer to 2,385) by keeping protein steady and modestly reducing carbohydrate and fat intake.

Note that in addition to the items already mentioned, a diligent and consistent resistance training program will be required to gain muscle, which will be discussed later in this chapter.

3. Pick Your Macro Split

Given the scenarios, the following macro formulation for all three individuals is proposed, although there is flexibility for those who want more protein or fat and less carbohydrates, depending on food preferences. For those who wish to further modify their macronutrients, it's recommended that protein be kept at a minimum of 25 percent at all times.

Carbohydrates: 50 percent (or 5 to 10 percent lower)

Proteins: 25 percent (or 5 to 10 percent higher)

Fats: 25 percent (or 5 to 10 percent higher)

4. Calculate the Grams for Each Macro

Continuing the scenarios, and using the calculated macro formulations, let's calculate grams for each macro. Although these macro recommendations are solid starting points for each of the cases, the right number could vary significantly based on the starting point, personal characteristics, and medium-term goals.

Carbohydrates: 50 percent total and 4 calories per gram

Proteins: 25 percent total and 4 calories per gram

Fats: 25 percent total and 9 calories per gram

CASE #1: 2,350 CALORIES

Carbohydrates: 2,350 x 50% = 1175/4 = 294 grams carbohydrates

Proteins: 2,350 x 25% = 588/4 = 147 grams protein

Fats: 2,350 x 25% = 588/9 = 65 grams fat

CASE #2: 2,817 CALORIES

Carbohydrates: 2,817 x 50% = 1,409/4 = 352 grams carbohydrates

Proteins: 2,817 x 25% = 704/4 = 176 grams protein*

Fats: 2,817 x 25% = 704/9 = 78 grams fat

   *Note that this ends up surpassing my protein recommendation of .8 grams per lb., and so this individual could transfer some protein calories to carbohydrates or fat if they saw fit, or maintain as is.

CASE #3: 2,635 CALORIES

Carbohydrates: 2,635 x 50% = 1,318/4 = 330 grams carbohydrates

Proteins: 2,635 x 25% = 659/4 = 165 grams protein

Fats: 2,635 x 25% = 659/9 = 73 grams fat

   It's normal that modifications to these numbers may be needed after a trial period. The upcoming sections address how to adjust these numbers if the desired result isn't being achieved.

Choosing Foods That Work for You

Although there are wildly different ways to reach calorie, carbohydrate, fat, and protein daily goals, these macros aren't all equal in terms of their impact on health. The goal is to have 80 percent of your weekly caloric intake come from nutrient-dense foods that have other favorable characteristics, such as high fiber content, healthy fat content, and an abundance of antioxidants and other useful components.

That leaves 20 percent that can be used as seen fit. For example, if the daily caloric target is 2,000 calories, that equates to a total of 14,000 calories per week. At 20 percent, that leaves 2,800 weekly "free" calories. The remaining 80 percent will be derived from protein, which is what the next section is about.

Protein

Protein is a cornerstone of good health, and it can be placed into several categories:

Animal: chicken breast and thigh, eggs, lean ground beef/pork/poultry, pork tenderloin, eye of round

Plant: tofu, tempeh, soy milk, vegan meat products & legumes

Marine: all fish/seafood

Dairy: Greek yogurt and milk

Animal and marine sources provide more protein per gram consumed than plant and dairy sources.

Carbohydrates

Ideally, carbohydrates that contain significant amounts of dietary fiber are best, because it's often difficult to get enough fiber. The most nutrient-dense carbohydrates can be found in a few different families of foods:

Whole grains: brown rice, quinoa, whole-grain bread, oatmeal, cereal

Starchy vegetables: sweet potatoes, potatoes, squash, beets

Legumes: lentils, chickpeas, black beans (also a great source of protein)

Fruit

Fats

Regardless of fitness goals, I never recommend dropping fat intake lower than 20 percent of daily calories, because there is a substantial amount of nutritional value in fats. Key sources of the healthiest types of fats include:

Nuts and seeds

Fish: especially salmon, trout, and sardines

Avocado

Soy-based foods

For those who do not consume fish, it's important to know that the essential omega-3 fatty acid found in fish can also be found in flaxseed, chia seed, hempseed, and walnuts.

Micronutrients (Vitamins and Minerals)

Micronutrients are the various vitamins and minerals found in food. Vitamins are vital for energy production, immune function, determining where minerals help with growth, bone health, and other processes. If fish, nuts, vegetables, legumes, and fruits make up 80 percent of your diet, in addition to protein or starchy foods from the sources previously discussed, it is highly unlikely there will be a micronutrient deficiency. The biggest exception to this rule is for omnivores who don't eat fish, so they may need a vitamin D supplement to make up for it. Vegans and vegetarians may also have unique challenges when it comes to certain key nutrients, such as iron and vitamin B_{12}.

Beyond micronutrients, there are also compounds known as phytochemicals, which are antioxidants mostly found in plant-based foods. Different varieties of food, especially varying colors of fruits and vegetables, contain different types of unique and healthy phytochemicals, which justifies the "eat the rainbow" concept. Tomatoes, for example, contain lycopene, which may protect against prostate cancer, certainly a very relevant consideration for men's health.

WHAT ABOUT BEVERAGES?

Fluid hydration is critically important, because hydration impacts body temperature regulation, infection prevention, nutrient delivery between cells, sleep quality, mood, and so much more. The official fluid recommendation for men is 3.7 liters of liquid daily, including incidental fluid intake from coffee, tea, and the water naturally present in food. Assuming that this incidental consumption amounts to more than a liter of water per day, the recommended amount of pure water for consumption is around 2.5 liters daily.

Things like coffee could either have no impact or could contribute significantly to hydration levels; it depends on the type of beverage. A premade mixed drink from a coffee shop, for example, could have 400 calories, whereas a small black coffee might only have 4 calories. Sugar-sweetened beverages and alcohol, depending on the variety and amount, also contribute calories and must be taken into consideration toward daily totals. For example, a can of beer, soda, or a glass of wine will contribute about 125 to 150 calories per serving, so do keep this in mind.

Planning for Success

The following sections provide tips and insights on pulling together everything discussed so far. Meal planning, prepping, and tracking progress are all effective tools for reaching macro goals. The key is knowing the options and working with what is most comfortable.

Meal Planning

The large library of recipes in this book provides a strong foundation to begin this journey. Meal planning is determining how to best approach the recipes. The more variety, the more ingredients and prep time needed. Most recipes include variation tips, so don't be timid. An alternative approach, and one many of my clients prefer, is having a few select meals they use over and over again. This certainly brings a level of simplicity to the program. If there are a few recipes that stand out above the rest, rotate through them every week.

The recipes are created so that they may be easily combined and modified. Be aware that it's important to maintain weekly and monthly diversity so that all the key food groups discussed in the previous section are eaten.

My clients often ask me about weighing food, especially those who enjoy being very precise in their plans. It's really up to the individual and not a requirement. Estimating serving sizes with measuring cups is usually good enough.

Meal Prepping

People who cook tend to fall into one of two categories: the individual who will spend their Sunday shopping and prepping for the week or the individual who will cook dinner each night and use the leftovers for lunch the next day.

The Sunday shopper is the best method for those who don't want to think about cooking during the week, but the repetitiveness of the meals may or may not be appealing to some. The nightly cook can have either the lunch or dinner recipes for dinner and a daily variety with fresher meals. The disadvantage with this approach is the nightly cooking, which may be more time consuming. Beginners should try both methods to determine preference, but keep in mind, lifestyle changes like holidays and changes in work schedules may impact which works best.

Tracking and Troubleshooting Progress

The advantage of having a scheduled meal plan is that it reduces the burden of tracking macros. Once the meal plan is expanded and more diverse options are added, it becomes more important to understand macro content in food.

Keep in mind that even in following this book, there are unknown variables that are difficult to plan or control for, such as genetics, current muscle mass, and energy level possibilities at any time. As a result, there is always the chance that a macro calculation won't be perfectly suitable on the first attempt. With that in mind, a two-week settling period with the macro configuration is important before assessing effectiveness. Try the plan for at least two weeks before making any changes.

80/20 IN PRACTICE

Although the 80/20 rule may be the ultimate nutrition cliché, it is something that resonates with many people. It allows for flexibility, which is important because it aids in long-term stickiness with the program. If a program is too rigid, people tend to drop it. Pursuing muscle strength, increasing muscle mass, and working on body composition is a medium-term endeavor that requires a long-term commitment to sustain.

Implementing the 80/20 mindset is a personal choice. Looking at it broadly, someone trying to add serious muscle by eating 4,000 calories a day would consume 28,000 calories over a 7-day period. If they choose the 80/20 approach to their macros, 20 percent of 28,000 is 5,600 calories. This individual now has 5,600 "free" calories per week to consume as they see fit. They could, of course, consume all 5,600 on one day and then control their intake on the subsequent days.

Tracking "free" calories is a personal choice, but it is helpful in breaking the monotony of a routine and does help facilitate a normal social life, both of which are important considerations for long-term success.

Combining Food and Fitness

Physical activity has a significant role in maintaining good health. This is especially true for those with muscle-gain goals, which simply cannot be facilitated without consistent and well-planned resistance training.

Fat-loss goals can be achieved by incorporating exercise into the plan because exercise increases energy expenditure and stimulates muscle growth while also improving so many other parameters of physical and mental health. According to a 2014 article by Damon Swift, studies show that exercise programs are much more effective at fat loss when paired with a proper nutrition program.

Fat Loss

A strategic approach to nutrition can be complemented by the inclusion of various types of physical activity, although some may be more efficient than others when it comes to promoting fat loss. It takes twice the amount of time to expend the same amount of energy via moderate-intensity cardio (like running) versus HIIT-based workouts. In a 2017 study by Haifeng Zhang in the *Journal for Diabetes Research*, researchers found that it actually took 60 minutes of moderate cardio to match the caloric expenditure of only 30 minutes of HIIT. A 2020 study in the journal *Medicine & Science in Sports & Exercise* found that, when it comes to losing fat, performing HIIT only once a week may be as effective as three weekly sessions of traditional aerobic cardiovascular activity.

Muscle Gain

Resistance training is the cornerstone of any muscle-gain program, and it's easily fueled by the additional energy found with a macro-focused nutritional plan. Resistance-based workouts completed multiple times a week that emphasize different body parts and include increasing difficulty are also an important part of muscle growth.

Cardio and HIIT-related activities on non-resistance days will offer health benefits and keep aerobic fitness strong; however, a weekly routine should emphasize resistance training.

General Tips

Take it from someone who built their fitness from a standing start; these quick workout tips are invaluable.

Warm up and cool down: It's easy to overlook the value of a proper warm up and cool down routine, but these types of considerations have a massive role to play in improving performance and preventing injury in the long term.

Strategize your routine: Plan a weekly routine that puts the best foot forward each exercise session. Don't put four resistance days back-to-back if by day three the soreness will prevent you from working out effectively.

Start slow, finish strong: In the grand scheme of things, fitness is a journey. If new to a regular workout program, know that this is a medium-term endeavor, and you should ease in slowly, gradually pushing harder over time as capacity increases.

Getting Started with the Meal Plans

In chapter 2, there are three 7-day meal plans at different calorie levels that align with different goals: fat loss, muscle gain, and an approach that favors neither.

Fat Loss

People who are pursuing fat loss typically do so because either they feel they are carrying significantly more body fat than they are comfortable with, or they haven't developed a desire to gain more muscle mass yet. When the right macronutrient and caloric targets are complemented by physical training, it is possible to lose between 0.5 to 1 pound of body fat or more on a weekly basis.

To facilitate this goal, reduce calorie intake by 500 calories per day. This number is only an estimate and may need to be modified after a 1- to 2-week test period. The macro split used for fat loss in this book is 50 percent carbohydrates/25 percent fat/25 percent protein, although going slightly higher in protein and a touch lower in fat or carbohydrates is acceptable. This will create a stronger satiating effect from the protein intake, which is helpful when consuming less calories than normal. Emphasizing legume-based meals (lentils, chickpeas, etc.), which are high in both protein and fiber, is a smart way to improve satiety.

Muscle Gain

The muscle-gain plan is recommended for those with a primary goal of adding size in the form of muscle mass. Use the 50/25/25 macro split, which facilitates sufficient protein intake for muscle gain while allowing for flexibility in proper nutrition across the other macronutrients.

Five hundred calories have been added to the baseline energy expenditure calculation. This additional calorie intake is supported by regular resistance training, which should stimulate muscle growth at the rate of about 0.25 to 0.5 pound per week in beginners. This approach will encourage a slow and steady gain, which ensures mostly lean mass being added. Note that if weight increases too quickly, the numbers may need to be modified.

Maintenance

If neither fat loss nor muscle gain is the priority, calories have been kept at a level for weight maintenance. If slight fat loss is a priority, reduce the calorie count by 250 calories, given that the body has potential to lose fat more quickly than it does to gain muscle.

It is possible for individuals who are new to physical training to lose fat and gain muscle simultaneously while maintaining, or slightly dropping, body weight. Combining resistance training with either HIIT or cardio in equal measure is a good approach to accomplish this.

Maintaining Your Results

Body composition goals tend to be dynamic and change over time. Changing body composition in a meaningful way is also a medium-term endeavor. This means that once the macro content level is achieved, it's very likely that these will be the numbers used for multiple months going forward. As body goals and training change over time, more significant changes may be required. Whether the numbers need to go up or down will depend on a variety of factors, but it's strongly recommended that protein is kept at a constant minimum of about 0.75 grams of protein per pound, or 1.6 gram per kilogram, of body weight.

FAT LOSS VS. MUSCLE GAIN RECIPE LABELS

Included with every recipe is one of two labels: **fat loss** or **muscle gain**. These labels are a guide to help determine which recipes work best for which goals. In general, fat-loss recipes are higher in protein, whereas muscle-gain recipes include more calories.

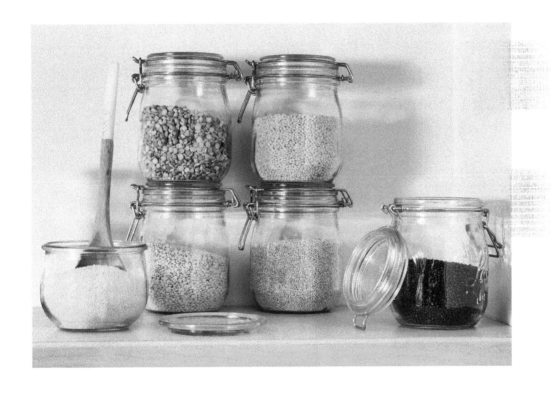

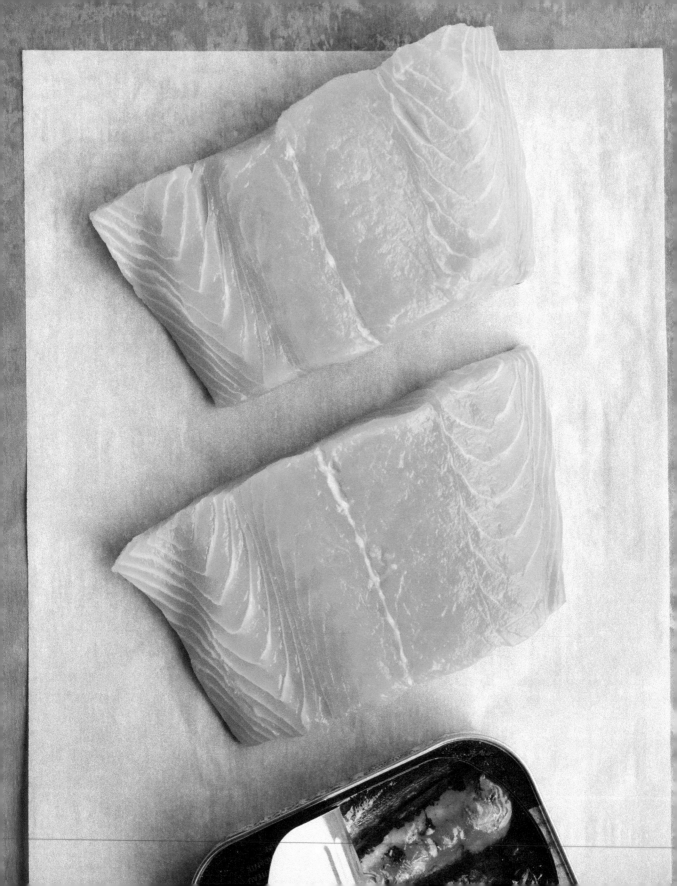

CHAPTER 2

7-DAY MEAL PLANS FOR FAT LOSS AND MUSCLE GAIN

This chapter includes three types of meal and exercise plans: fat loss, muscle gain, and fat loss with muscle gain. All three meal plans are designed for one person and include a chart outlining a week's worth of meals and snacks and a recommended workout. In addition, each chart includes a shopping list for that week and meal prep advice. In developing these plans, the goal was to keep things simple by reusing ingredients, maximizing leftovers, and keeping food waste to a minimum.

7-Day Fat-Loss Meal and Exercise Plan

In addition to the daily meals, the minimum expectation is three to four workouts weekly. On rest days, feel free to do mobility or resistance training. Prep-ahead information can be found on page 32.

BREAKFAST	SNACK	LUNCH	SNACK	DINNER
MONDAY				
WORKOUT: HIIT/Cardio				
Broccoli and Cheese Frittata (page 42) with whole-grain toast and fruit	Apple and 1 tablespoon nut butter	Salmon-Avocado Lettuce Wraps (page 91)	2 hard-boiled eggs and ½ avocado	Bean and Pumpkin Stew (page 63)
TUESDAY				
WORKOUT: Rest/Mobility or Resistance workout				
Leftover Broccoli and Cheese Frittata tucked in a tortilla	¼ cup roasted almonds	*Leftover Salmon-Avocado Lettuce Wraps*	Apple and 1 tablespoon nut butter	Sirloin and Bok Choy Stir-Fry (page 101)
WEDNESDAY				
WORKOUT: HIIT/Cardio				
Lemon-Blueberry Baked Oatmeal Cups (page 48) with fresh fruit (2 cups)	2 hard-boiled eggs	*Leftover Bean and Pumpkin Stew*	Mixed vegetables with 2 tablespoons low-fat dressing	*Leftover Sirloin and Bok Choy Stir-Fry*

	BREAKFAST	SNACK	LUNCH	SNACK	DINNER
THURSDAY					
WORKOUT: Rest/Mobility or Resistance workout					
	Leftover Lemon-Blueberry Baked Oatmeal Cups	2 hard-boiled eggs	*Leftover Sirloin and Bok Choy Stir-Fry*	½ cup Greek yogurt topped with blueberries	Bruschetta Chicken (page 92)
FRIDAY					
WORKOUT: HIIT/Cardio					
	Leftover Broccoli and Cheese Frittata with whole-grain toast and fruit	Apple with 1 tablespoon nut butter	*Leftover Bean and Pumpkin Stew*	*Leftover Lemon-Blueberry Baked Oatmeal Cups*	*Leftover Bruschetta Chicken*
SATURDAY					
WORKOUT: Rest/Mobility or Resistance workout					
	Leftover Lemon-Blueberry Baked Oatmeal Cups	*Leftover Broccoli and Cheese Frittata*	Spinach, Chicken, and Lentil Salad (page 85)	Mixed vegetables with 2 tablespoons low-fat dressing	Reader's choice
SUNDAY					
WORKOUT: HIIT/Cardio					
	Egg-Topped Sweet Potato Toast (page 50)	*Leftover Lemon-Blueberry Baked Oatmeal Cups*	*Leftover Spinach, Chicken, and Lentil Salad*	Mixed vegetables with 2 tablespoons low-fat dressing	Reader's choice

Shopping List

PRODUCE

- Apples (3)
- Avocado, ripe (1)
- Basil, fresh (1 bunch)
- Bell peppers, red (2)
- Blueberries (2 pints)
- Bok choy, baby (20)
- Broccoli (1 bunch)
- Carrots (2)
- Celery (1 bunch)
- Cucumber, English (1)
- Garlic, minced (1 head)
- Green beans (3 cups)
- Lemon (1)
- Lettuce (1 head)
- Lime (1)
- Mixed fruit (desired amount)
- Mixed vegetables (desired amount)
- Onions, red (1) and sweet (2)
- Scallions (1 bunch)
- Spinach, baby (3 [5-ounce] bags)
- Sweet potato (1)
- Tomatoes, large (6)

DAIRY, EGGS, AND NONDAIRY ALTERNATIVES

- Almond milk, unsweetened (1 quart)
- Cheese, cheddar, shredded (1 [6-ounce] bag)
- Cheese, Parmesan, shredded (1 [4-ounce] container)
- Eggs, large (2 dozen)
- Yogurt, Greek, plain (1 [17.6-ounce] container)

MEAT AND SEAFOOD

- Beef, steak, sirloin (12 ounces)
- Chicken, cooked (1½ cups) *1 rotisserie chicken
- Chicken, breasts, boneless, skinless (8 ounces)

FROZEN

- Edamame, frozen (1 [12-ounce] bag)
- Pumpkin, fresh or frozen (2 [10-ounce] bags)

HERBS AND SPICES

- Cinnamon, ground
- Italian seasoning
- Oregano, dried
- Peppercorns, black
- Sea salt
- Thyme, dried

PANTRY

- Almonds, roasted (¼ cup)
- Baking powder
- Beans, great northern, no-salt-added (2 [15-ounce] cans)
- Broth, beef, low-sodium (1 [15-ounce] can)
- Broth, chicken, low-sodium (1 [15-ounce] can)
- Broth, vegetable, low-sodium (2 [32-ounce] containers)
- Chickpeas, no-salt-added (1 [15-ounce] can)
- Cooking spray, nonstick
- Cornstarch
- Couscous, whole wheat (1 cup)
- Flaxseed, ground (2 tablespoons)
- Lentils, no-salt-added (3 [15-ounce] cans)
- Maple syrup
- Nut butter
- Oats, rolled (4 cups)
- Oil, olive
- Oil, sesame
- Salad dressing, balsamic, low-fat
- Salad dressing, low-fat
- Salmon, water-packed, boneless (2 [5-ounce] cans)
- Soy sauce, low-sodium
- Vanilla extract
- Vinegar, balsamic

OTHER

- Bread, whole-grain (1 loaf)
- Protein powder, plain, vegan (1 [12-ounce] container)
- Tortillas (1 pack)

7-Day Muscle-Gain Meal and Exercise Plan

Choose to do resistance workouts either three or six days a week; the following option is for six days. If three days are preferred (which is ideal for beginners), intersperse rest/cardio/HIIT and mobility workouts (similar to the plan on page 28). Prep-ahead information can be found on page 32.

BREAKFAST	SNACK	LUNCH	SNACK	DINNER
MONDAY				
WORKOUT: Resistance workout (push)				
Chocolate Granola (page 46; 1½ servings) with milk or nondairy milk	Carrots and cherry tomatoes with ¼ cup hummus	Two-Bean Veggie Salad (page 67)	Apple with 1 tablespoon almond or peanut butter	Creamy Corn Chowder (page 75) with a mixed green salad or slice of whole-grain bread
TUESDAY				
WORKOUT: Resistance workout (pull)				
Berry Smoothie Bowl (page 37; double recipe, and consume 1 serving)	Carrots and cherry tomatoes with ¼ cup hummus	*Leftover Two-Bean Veggie Salad*	*Leftover Chocolate Granola topping ½ cup Greek yogurt*	Sheet Pan Salmon with Mixed Vegetables (page 89)
WEDNESDAY				
WORKOUT: Resistance workout (legs)				
Leftover Berry Smoothie Bowl	*Leftover Creamy Corn Chowder (½ portion)*	*Leftover Sheet Pan Salmon with Mixed Vegetables*	Celery with 1 tablespoon almond or peanut butter	Black Bean Veggie Burgers (page 64)

BREAKFAST	SNACK	LUNCH	SNACK	DINNER
THURSDAY				
WORKOUT: Rest/Cardio/HIIT/Mobility workout				
Easy Tofu Scramble (page 43) in a whole wheat tortilla with salsa and a couple tablespoons shredded cheese	Carrots and cherry tomatoes with ¼ cup hummus	*Leftover Black Bean Veggie Burgers*	*Leftover Creamy Corn Chowder (½ portion)*	Speedy Beef Stroganoff (page 98)
FRIDAY				
WORKOUT: Resistance workout (push)				
Leftover Easy Tofu Scramble with whole-grain toast and sliced tomato	*Leftover Chocolate Granola*	*Leftover Creamy Corn Chowder* with a whole-grain bun	Apple with 1 tablespoon almond or peanut butter	*Leftover Speedy Beef Stroganoff*
SATURDAY				
WORKOUT: Resistance workout (pull)				
Leftover Chocolate Granola (1½ servings) with milk or nondairy milk	Celery with 1 tablespoon almond or peanut butter	*Leftover Speedy Beef Stroganoff*	Apple with 1 tablespoon almond or peanut butter	Reader's choice
SUNDAY				
WORKOUT: Resistance workout (legs)				
Leftover Chocolate Granola (1½ servings) with milk or nondairy milk	Carrots and cherry tomatoes with ¼ cup hummus	*Leftover Speedy Beef Stroganoff*	Celery with 1 tablespoon almond or peanut butter	Reader's choice

Shopping List

PRODUCE

- Apples (3)
- Berries, any (1 pint)
- Broccoli (1 bunch)
- Carrots (5)
- Cauliflower (1 head)
- Celery (1 bunch)
- Cucumber, English (1)
- Garlic (1 head)
- Lemon (1)
- Mushrooms, white (10 ounces)
- Onions, sweet (3)
- Parsley (1 bunch)
- Parsnips (2)
- Potatoes (2)
- Scallion (1 bunch)
- Sweet potato (1)
- Thyme, fresh (1 bunch)
- Tomato (1)
- Tomatoes, cherry (3 pints)

DAIRY, EGGS, AND NONDAIRY ALTERNATIVES

- Almond milk, unsweetened (1 quart)
- Cheese, any, shredded (1 [6-ounce] bag)
- Cheese, feta (1 [4-ounce] container)
- Cheese, Swiss, low-fat (4 slices)
- Eggs, large (½ dozen)
- Sour cream, full-fat (1 [8-ounce] container)
- Tofu, firm (1 [14-ounce] block)
- Yogurt, Greek, plain (1 [7-ounce] container)

MEAT AND SEAFOOD

- Bacon (8 slices)
- Beef, steak, sirloin (12 ounces)
- Salmon, skinless (2 [6-ounce] fillets)

FROZEN

- Corn, fresh or frozen (½ cup)
- Edamame, fresh or frozen (1 [12-ounce] bag)
- Strawberries, unsweetened, frozen (1 [10-ounce] bag)

HERBS AND SPICES

- Cumin, ground (2 teaspoons)
- Sea salt
- Peppercorns, black
- Turmeric (½ teaspoon)

PANTRY

- Almonds, ground (⅓ cup)
- Almonds, slivered or sliced (¾ cup)
- Beans, black, no-salt-added (2 [15-ounce] cans)
- Beans, kidney, no-salt-added (1 [15-ounce] can)
- Broth, beef, low-sodium (1 [15-ounce] can)
- Broth, vegetable, low-sodium (1 [32-ounce] container)
- Cocoa powder, unsweetened
- Corn, creamed, no-salt-added (2 [15-ounce] cans)
- Egg noodles, whole wheat (8 ounces)
- Flour, all-purpose
- Maple syrup
- Mustard, Dijon
- Nut butter
- Oats, rolled (4 cups)
- Oil, avocado
- Oil, coconut
- Oil, olive
- Salsa
- Salad dressing, balsamic, low-fat
- Seeds, chia (2 tablespoons)
- Seeds, pumpkin (½ cup)
- Seeds, sesame (2 tablespoons)
- Seeds, sunflower (½ cup)
- Vanilla extract
- Worcestershire sauce

OTHER

- Bread, whole-grain (1 loaf)
- Buns, whole wheat (4)
- Hummus (1 [10-ounce] container)
- Nutritional yeast
- Protein powder, chocolate (1 [12-ounce] container)
- Protein powder, unsweetened, vegan (1 [12-ounce] container)
- Tortillas, whole wheat (1 pack)

7-Day Muscle-Gain and Fat-Loss Meal and Exercise Plan

The following is based on three days a week of resistance training interspersed with cardio/HIIT/mobility. If a more resistance-heavy routine is preferred, see the workout schedule in the previous plan. Prep-ahead information can be found on page 33.

BREAKFAST	SNACK	LUNCH	SNACK	DINNER
MONDAY				
WORKOUT: Resistance workout (push)				
Peanut Butter and Strawberry Overnight Oats (page 47)	Cut mixed vegetables with low-fat dressing	Classic Chicken Noodle Soup (page 83)	Zucchini-Banana Muffins (page 49; 1 muffin)	Cheeseburger Bowls (page 100)
TUESDAY				
WORKOUT: Cardio/HIIT/Mobility workout				
Loaded Breakfast Casserole (page 45)	*Leftover Zucchini-Banana Muffins (1 muffin)*	*Leftover Cheeseburger Bowls*	Cut mixed vegetables with low-fat dressing	Caprese Turkey Burgers (page 77) with a mixed green salad
WEDNESDAY				
WORKOUT: Resistance workout (pull)				
Leftover Peanut Butter and Strawberry Overnight Oats	½ cup Greek yogurt	*Leftover Cheeseburger Bowls*	*Leftover Zucchini-Banana Muffins (1 muffin)*	*Leftover Caprese Turkey Burgers with a mixed green salad*

	BREAKFAST	SNACK	LUNCH	SNACK	DINNER

| **THURSDAY** |

WORKOUT: Cardio/HIIT/Mobility workout

	BREAKFAST	SNACK	LUNCH	SNACK	DINNER
	Leftover Peanut Butter and Strawberry Overnight Oats	Leftover Zucchini-Banana Muffins (1 muffin)	Leftover Classic Chicken Noodle Soup	Leftover Loaded Breakfast Casserole (½ serving)	Leftover Caprese Turkey Burgers with a mixed green salad

| **FRIDAY** |

WORKOUT: Resistance workout (legs)

	BREAKFAST	SNACK	LUNCH	SNACK	DINNER
	Leftover Loaded Breakfast Casserole	Apple with 1 tablespoon nut butter	Leftover Classic Chicken Noodle Soup	Leftover Zucchini-Banana Muffins (1 muffin)	Pork, Winter Squash, and Cranberry Sauté (page 94)

| **SATURDAY** |

WORKOUT: Cardio/HIIT/Mobility workout

	BREAKFAST	SNACK	LUNCH	SNACK	DINNER
	Leftover Zucchini- Banana Muffins (1 muffin) with nut butter	Leftover Loaded Breakfast Casserole (½ serving)	Leftover Caprese Turkey Burgers	Cut mixed vegetables with low-fat dressing	Reader's choice

| **SUNDAY** |

WORKOUT: Rest

	BREAKFAST	SNACK	LUNCH	SNACK	DINNER
	Leftover Zucchini-Banana Muffins (1 muffin) with nut butter	¼ cup roasted almonds	Leftover Pork, Winter Squash, and Cranberry Sauté	Cut mixed vegetables with low-fat dressing	Reader's choice

Shopping List

PRODUCE

- Apple (1)
- Banana (1)
- Bell pepper, red (1)
- Broccoli (1 bunch)
- Brussels sprouts (1 pound)
- Carrots (3)
- Celery (1 bunch)
- Cranberries (1 [12-ounce] bag)
- Garlic (1 head)
- Leek (1)
- Lettuce, romaine (1 large head or 3 hearts)
- Mixed greens, any (2 [5-ounce] containers)
- Mixed vegetables, any (desired amount)
- Mushrooms, white (10 medium)
- Onion, sweet (1)
- Parsley, fresh (1 bunch)
- Scallions (1 bunch)
- Squash, winter (1 large)
- Strawberries (1 pint)
- Sweet potato (1 large)
- Tomatoes (3)
- Zucchini (3)

DAIRY, EGGS, AND NONDAIRY ALTERNATIVES

- Almond milk, unsweetened (1 quart)
- Cheese, cheddar, shredded (1 [6-ounce] bag)
- Cheese, mozzarella, low-fat (4 slices)
- Eggs, large (1 dozen)
- Yogurt, Greek, plain (1 [17.6-ounce] container)

MEAT AND SEAFOOD

- Beef, ground, extra-lean (12 ounces)
- Chicken, cooked (2 cups) *1 rotisserie chicken
- Pork, ground, extra-lean (12 ounces)
- Turkey, ground, extra-lean (1 pound)

HERBS AND SPICES

- Cinnamon, ground
- Nutmeg, ground
- Oregano, dried
- Paprika
- Peppercorns, black
- Sea salt
- Thyme, dried

PANTRY

- Almonds, roasted (¼ cup)
- Baking powder
- Bread crumbs
- Broth, chicken, low-sodium (2 [32-ounce] containers)
- Cooking spray, nonstick
- Egg noodles, thin soup (1 [12-ounce] bag)
- Flaxseed, ground (½ cup)
- Flour, oat (1 cup)
- Lentils, low-sodium (2 [15-ounce] cans)
- Maple syrup
- Nut butter
- Oats, rolled (3 cups)
- Oil, olive
- Peanut butter, natural
- Pesto, basil
- Pickles, sweet
- Salad dressing, ranch or honey mustard, low-fat
- Vanilla extract

OTHER

- Bread, whole-grain (1 loaf)
- Buns, hamburger, whole wheat (4)
- Protein powder, plain, vegan or unsweetened whey (1 [12-ounce] container)

Prep Ahead: Fat-Loss Plan

- Make the Broccoli and Cheese Frittata (page 42), and store 2 portions in the refrigerator and 2 portions in the freezer. Take the frozen portion out the day before it is needed, and thaw in the refrigerator.

- Make the Lemon-Blueberry Baked Oatmeal Cups (page 48), and freeze them in plastic sealable bags (2 per bag). Take them out the night before serving, and thaw in the refrigerator.

- Make the Bean and Pumpkin Stew (page 63), place 2 portions in the refrigerator, and freeze 1 portion. Take the portion out to thaw in the refrigerator the day before serving.

- Hard-boil 6 eggs and store in the refrigerator.

Prep Ahead: Muscle-Gain Plan

- Prep the double recipe of the base of the Berry Smoothie Bowl (page 37), divide between 2 containers, and store in the refrigerator.

- Make the Chocolate Granola (page 46), and refrigerate in a container.

- Make the Speedy Beef Stroganoff (page 98), and store 2 portions in the refrigerator and 2 in the freezer. Take out the frozen portions the night before serving, and thaw in the refrigerator.

- Make the Creamy Corn Chowder (page 75), and separate into 2 full portions and 2 half portions. Keep 1 full portion out, and freeze the other 3 containers. Take the frozen portions out the night before serving, and thaw in the refrigerator.

- Make the Two-Bean Veggie Salad (page 67), and refrigerate the 2 portions.

Prep Ahead: Muscle-Gain and Fat-Loss Plan

- Make the Peanut Butter and Strawberry Overnight Oats (page 47), and store all 3 portions in the refrigerator. Stir before eating.

- Make the Zucchini-Banana Muffins (page 49), and freeze in a container or plastic freezer bags. Take the required muffins out the night before, and thaw at room temperature.

- Make the Classic Chicken Noodle Soup (page 83), and store 1 portion in the refrigerator and 2 in the freezer. Take the frozen portions out the night before serving, and thaw in the refrigerator.

- Make the Loaded Breakfast Casserole (page 45), and store 1 portion in the refrigerator and 1 full portion and 2 half portions in the freezer. Take the frozen portions out the night before serving, and thaw in the refrigerator

- Optional: Make the Caprese Turkey Burgers (page 77) patties, and freeze them raw between pieces of parchment paper. Take the patties out, and thaw in the refrigerator overnight. Cook them on the first day used in the meal plan, and store the cooked patties in the refrigerator for up to 4 days.

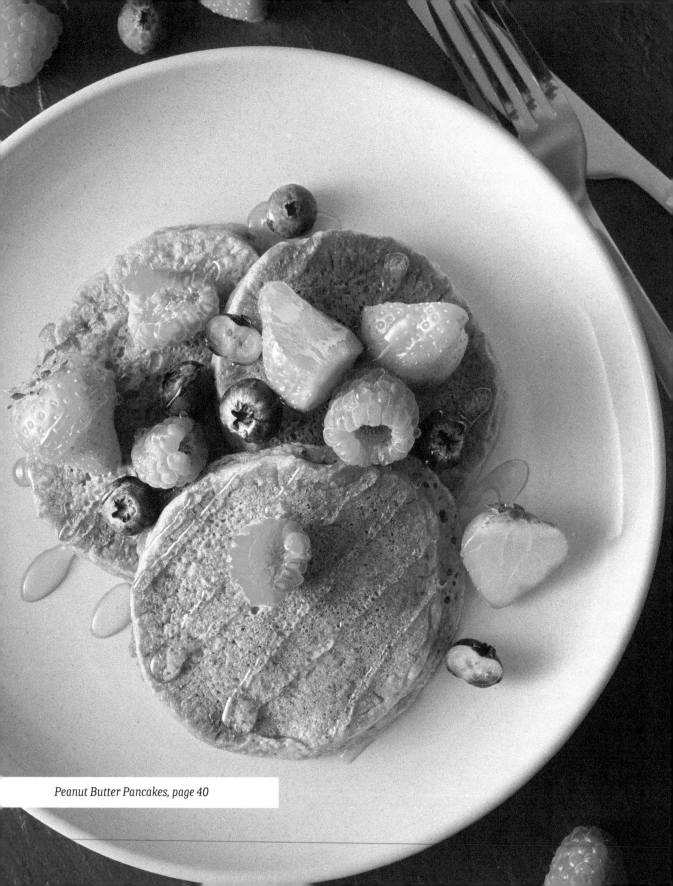

Peanut Butter Pancakes, page 40

BREAKFAST

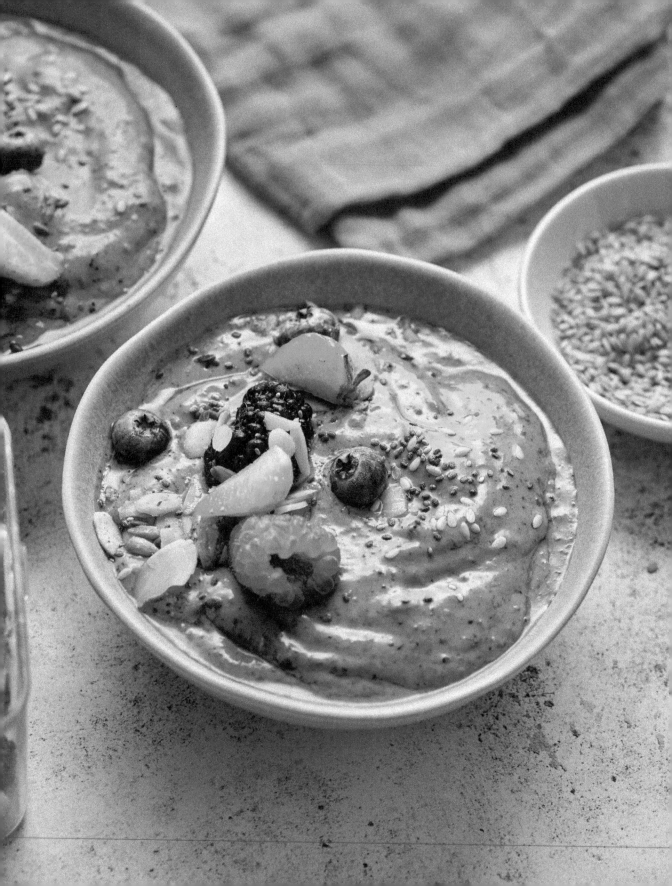

Berry Smoothie Bowl

PREP TIME: 10 minutes | Serves 1 | **MUSCLE GAIN**

Smoothies are not just beverages; they can also be enjoyed like a meal with a spoon, full of healthy toppings. The benefit of this presentation is the marvelous texture from the nuts, fruit, and seeds that would instead be pureed if this were a standard smoothie. Try whatever suits the palate, such as avocado, sunflower seeds, hemp hearts, or a couple tablespoons of granola.

1 cup frozen strawberries

½ cup unsweetened almond milk

1 scoop unsweetened vegan (or regular) protein powder

1 teaspoon pure vanilla extract

½ cup fresh berries, such as blueberries, raspberries, and strawberries

2 tablespoons sliced or slivered almonds

1 tablespoon chia seeds

1 tablespoon sesame seeds

1. Put the strawberries, almond milk, protein powder, and vanilla in a blender. Pulse until the mixture is smooth. Transfer to a bowl.

2. Top with the berries, almonds, chia seeds, and sesame seeds.

FAT-LOSS TIP: Add more fresh fruit, and omit the seeds from the smoothie. This will drop the fat by 10 grams, the protein by 3 grams, and the carbohydrates by 6 grams. The macros will be 34 percent protein, 26 percent fat, and 40 percent carbohydrates.

PER SERVING: Calories: 507; Protein: 32g; Total carbohydrates: 51g; Fiber: 13g; Fat: 20g

MACROS: 26% Protein; 34% Fat; 40% Carbohydrates=

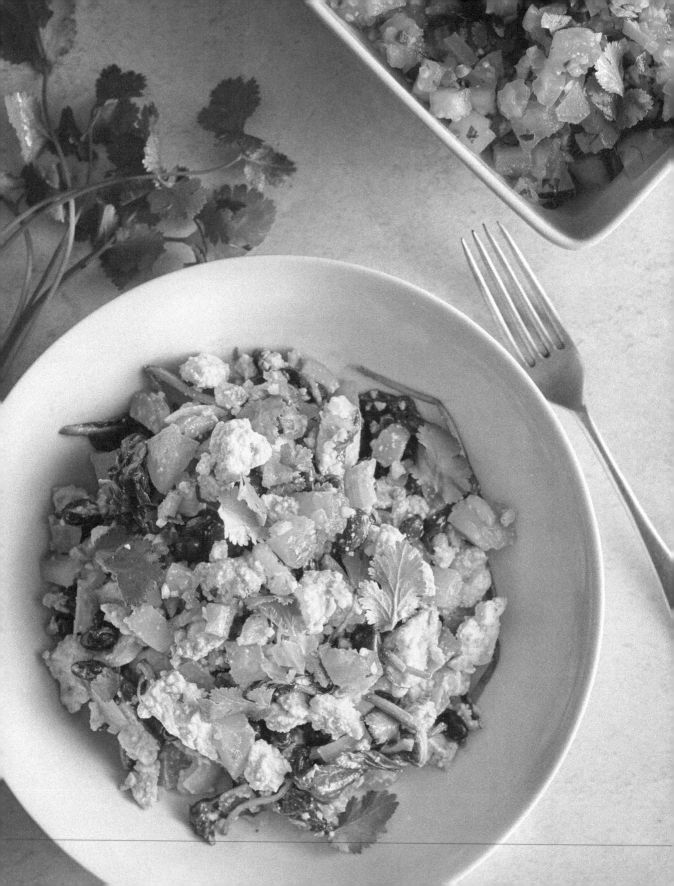

Southwest Scrambled Eggs

PREP TIME: 10 minutes | COOK TIME: 10 minutes | Serves 3 | FAT LOSS

Scrambled eggs are often thought to be a bland but healthy dish, but packing them with color-ful vegetables, spices, and herbs creates a flavorful meal. Enjoy them with fresh fruit or a slice of whole-grain toast. Throw in a pinch or two of turmeric for additional flavor and a festive, bright color.

5 large eggs

3 large egg whites

¼ cup 1 percent milk

½ teaspoon ground cumin

Sea salt

Freshly ground black pepper

2 teaspoons salted butter

¼ sweet onion, chopped

1 (15-ounce) can black beans, drained and rinsed

1 large tomato, chopped

1 cup baby spinach

2 tablespoons chopped fresh cilantro

1. In a large bowl, whisk together the eggs, egg whites, milk, and cumin until combined. Season with salt and pepper.

2. In a large skillet, melt the butter over medium heat.

3. Add the onion, and sauté for about 3 minutes, or until softened.

4. Pour in the egg mixture, and gently drag a spatula across the skillet, creating fluffy curds. Continue scrambling for about 5 minutes, or until the eggs are about three-quarters cooked (moist with some liquid).

5. Add the beans, tomato, and spinach. Fold for about 2 minutes, or until the eggs have thoroughly cooked and the spinach has wilted. Remove from the heat.

6. Serve the eggs topped with the cilantro. Refrigerate any leftovers in a sealed container for up to 3 days.

MUSCLE-GAIN TIP: Add 1 cup shredded cooked chicken—either leftovers or a store-bought rotisserie chicken—to the dish or an extra cup of beans to boost the protein by 13 grams per serving.

PER SERVING: Calories: 303; Protein: 24g; Total carbohydrates: 28g; Fiber: 9g; Fat: 11g
MACROS: 32% Protein; 33% Fat; 35% Carbohydrates

Peanut Butter Pancakes

PREP TIME: 10 minutes | COOK TIME: 25 minutes | Serves 4 | **FAT LOSS**

Pancakes are often the choice for special meals, a decadent treat drizzled in maple syrup. These peanut butter beauties are high in protein and freeze beautifully. They make for a delicious cold snack with a bit of strawberry jam.

2 large eggs

¼ cup peanut butter

½ teaspoon pure vanilla extract

½ cup almond flour

½ cup whole wheat flour

2 scoops vegan or unsweetened whey protein powder

1 teaspoon baking powder

Sea salt

Butter or nonstick cooking spray, for coating the skillet

1½ cups berries, such as raspberries, blueberries, or strawberries

Drizzle of maple syrup, for serving

1. In a medium bowl, whisk together the eggs, peanut butter, and vanilla until smooth.

2. Whisk in the almond flour, whole wheat flour, protein powder, baking powder, and salt until well combined.

3. In a large skillet, melt the butter over medium heat.

4. Working in batches of about 3, pour the batter in ¼-cup measures into the skillet, and cook for 3 to 4 minutes, or until golden brown on the bottom and tiny bubbles on the surface pop. Flip the pancakes over, and cook for 2 minutes. Transfer to a plate, and repeat with the remaining batter. Turn off the heat.

5. Serve the pancakes with the berries and a drizzle of maple syrup. Refrigerate any leftovers in a sealed container for up to 4 days or freeze for up to 1 month.

MUSCLE-GAIN TIP: Serve these with a side of peameal or turkey bacon for a protein boost.

PER SERVING (3 PANCAKES): Calories: 439; Protein: 24g; Total carbohydrates: 49g; Fiber: 6g; Fat: 18g

MACROS: 22% Protein; 33% Fat; 45% Carbohydrates

Eggy Breakfast "Pizza"

PREP TIME: 10 minutes | COOK TIME: 10 minutes | Serves 2 | **FAT LOSS**

This is more of a thin omelet with popular pizza toppings than an authentic pizza; the eggy crust is higher in protein than a standard bread bottom. For a grab-and-go meal, roll these up like tortillas.

5 large eggs

2 tomatoes, chopped

1 tablespoon chopped fresh basil leaves

Freshly ground black pepper

Nonstick cooking spray, for coating the skillet

¼ small onion, chopped

1 teaspoon minced garlic

1 cup sliced black or green olives (optional)

½ cup jalapeños (optional)

1 cup mushrooms (optional)

¼ cup shredded mozzarella cheese

2 whole-grain pita bread rounds, toasted

1. Set the oven to broil.

2. In a medium bowl, whisk together the eggs, tomatoes, and basil until well mixed. Season with pepper.

3. Lightly coat a large skillet with cooking spray, and heat over medium-high heat.

4. Add the onion and garlic. Sauté for about 3 minutes, or until softened.

5. Add the olives (if using), jalapeños (if using), and mushrooms (if using). Sauté until heated through. Shake to evenly disperse the toppings.

6. Pour the egg mixture over the toppings, and cook for 3 minutes, or until set on the bottom.

7. Sprinkle the cheese over the eggs, and transfer the skillet to the oven. Broil for about 2 minutes, or until the omelet is golden brown and bubbling. Remove from the oven.

8. Serve the omelet on the pitas. Refrigerate any leftovers in a sealed container for up to 2 days.

MUSCLE-GAIN TIP: Add toppings such as ground beef, turkey bacon, turkey sausage, or chicken to create a protein-packed breakfast.

PER SERVING (½ RECIPE): Calories: 419; Protein: 26g; Total carbohydrates: 42g; Fiber: 6g; Fat: 16g

MACROS: 25% Protein; 35% Fat; 40% Carbohydrates

Broccoli and Cheese Frittata

PREP TIME: 10 minutes | COOK TIME: 20 minutes | Serves 4 | FAT LOSS

Frittata is a versatile dish, thicker than an omelet and without the crust of quiche. Broccoli and cheddar are a classic pairing, with the earthy cruciferous vegetable adding fiber and bright color to the dish. Frittata can be eaten hot or cold, by itself or tucked into a tortilla.

4 large eggs

8 large egg whites

Sea salt

Freshly ground black pepper

Nonstick cooking spray, for coating the skillet

¼ onion, chopped

1 teaspoon minced garlic

3 cups chopped broccoli

2 cups canned lentils, drained and rinsed

¼ cup shredded cheddar cheese

1. Preheat the oven to 400°F.

2. In a medium bowl, whisk together the eggs and egg whites. Season with salt and pepper.

3. Spray a large oven-safe skillet generously with nonstick cooking spray, and heat over medium heat.

4. Add the onion and garlic. Sauté for about 3 minutes, or until softened.

5. Pour in the egg mixture, and scatter the broccoli and lentils over. Cook for 2 minutes, or until the bottom is set.

6. Sprinkle the top with cheese. Remove from the heat.

7. Transfer the skillet to the oven, and bake for about 15 minutes, or until the frittata is golden and puffed. Remove from the oven. Serve. Refrigerate any leftovers in a sealed container for up to 4 days or freeze for up to 1 month.

MUSCLE-GAIN TIP: Swap out the egg whites for 4 large eggs, and add 1 cup crumbled cooked turkey sausage to boost the protein by 5 grams per portion.

PER SERVING (¼ FRITTATA): Calories: 284; Protein: 27g; Total carbohydrates: 28g; Fiber: 10g; Fat: 8g

MACROS: 36% Protein; 24% Fat; 40% Carbohydrates

Easy Tofu Scramble

PREP TIME: 5 minutes, plus 30 minutes to press the tofu | COOK TIME: 10 minutes
Serves 2 | **MUSCLE GAIN**

Nutritional yeast can be surprising with its cheesy flavor. If Himalayan black salt (kala namak) is available, try it in this recipe as well. It adds a distinctly eggy and delightful taste to the tofu.

1 (14-ounce) block firm tofu

1 teaspoon coconut oil or avocado oil

2 tablespoons nutritional yeast

½ teaspoon turmeric

¼ teaspoon sea salt

2 tablespoons unsweetened almond milk

1 scallion, green and white parts, chopped

1. Wrap the tofu block in a clean kitchen towel, place on a plate, and set a weight (another plate or a large can) on top for 30 minutes. Unwrap the tofu.

2. In a large skillet, heat the oil over medium heat.

3. Crumble in the tofu, and sauté for 2 to 3 minutes, or until light brown and heated through.

4. Sprinkle in the nutritional yeast, turmeric, and salt. Sauté for about 5 minutes, or until any purged liquid has evaporated.

5. Add the almond milk and scallion. Sauté for 2 minutes, or until the scallion is slightly softened. Remove from the heat. Serve. Refrigerate any leftovers in a sealed container for up to 2 days.

FAT-LOSS TIP: Reduce the portion to half, and add a couple cups of chopped vegetables to the scramble, sautéing them to tender-crisp with the tofu.

PER SERVING (½ RECIPE): Calories: 350; Protein: 34g; Total carbohydrates: 13g; Fiber: 6g; Fat: 18g
MACROS: 40% Protein; 45% Fat; 15% Carbohydrates

Skillet Steak, Eggs, and Bok Choy Breakfast

PREP TIME: 10 minutes | COOK TIME: 14 minutes | Makes 1 Servings | **MUSCLE GAIN**

Steak and eggs are a satisfying country-style breakfast that might seem like too much work. Feel free to add other favorites like tomatoes, bacon, or mushrooms.

1 (4-ounce) top sirloin steak, trimmed of fat

Sea salt

Freshly ground black pepper

1 tablespoon olive oil, divided

8 baby bok choy, halved and washed

1 teaspoon minced garlic

1 large egg

1 scallion, white and green parts, thinly sliced

1. Preheat the oven to 325°F.

2. Bring the steak to room temperature and lightly season both sides with salt and pepper.

3. Place a large ovenproof skillet over high heat until it starts to smoke. Sear the steak for 2 minutes on each side. Move the steak to the side of the skillet and drizzle with 1 teaspoon of olive oil. Add the baby bok choy to the other side of the skillet, lightly season with salt and pepper, and toss with 1 teaspoon of oil and the garlic.

4. Place the skillet in the oven and cook for 5 to 8 minutes depending on desired doneness (internal temperature for medium-rare is 120°F). Remove from the oven and let rest for 5 minutes.

5. While the steak is resting, heat the remaining oil in a small skillet over medium-high heat. Fry the egg until the white is set and edges lightly browned, about 2 minutes for sunny-side up.

6. Serve the steak with the bok choy and fried egg, topped with the scallion.

FAT-LOSS TIP: Increase the steak to 6 ounces or add another egg for a boost in satiating protein.

PER SERVING (1 RECIPE): Calories: 503; Protein: 33g; Total carbohydrates: 25g; Fiber: 9g; Fat: 30g
MACROS: 28% Protein, 56% Fat, 16% Carbs

Loaded Breakfast Casserole

PREP TIME: 15 minutes | COOK TIME: 35 minutes | Serves 4 | **FAT LOSS**

Casseroles are the ultimate savory comfort food, and, because they are usually one-pan preparations, they can be thrown together easily. The ingredients in this protein-packed recipe can be swapped out for whatever is in the refrigerator. Try ground beef, chicken chunks, chopped kale, cauliflower florets, parsnips, or russet potatoes.

Nonstick cooking spray, for coating the baking dish

2 cups shredded sweet potatoes

2 cups shredded Brussels sprouts

1 cup chopped mushrooms

1 cup chopped broccoli

1 red bell pepper, cored and chopped

½ cup chopped onion

6 large eggs

4 large egg whites

2 teaspoons dried oregano

Sea salt

Freshly ground black pepper

4 whole-grain toast slices

1. Preheat the oven to 375°F. Coat a 9-by-13-inch baking dish with cooking spray.

2. Spread the sweet potatoes, Brussels sprouts, mushrooms, broccoli, bell pepper, and onion out in the prepared baking dish.

3. In a medium bowl, whisk together the eggs, egg whites, and oregano. Season with salt and pepper.

4. Pour the egg mixture over the other ingredients, and tap the baking dish to disperse the eggs.

5. Transfer the baking dish to the oven, and bake for about 35 minutes, or until the eggs have cooked through and the casserole has lightly browned. Remove from the oven.

6. Serve the casserole with the toast. Refrigerate any leftovers in a sealed container for up to 4 days or freeze for up to 1 month.

MUSCLE-GAIN TIP: Add either 1 cup shredded cheese, 1 cup cooked sausage, or shredded chicken to the casserole to boost calories, protein, and fat.

PER SERVING (¼ CASSEROLE): Calories: 308; Protein: 24g; Total carbohydrates: 34g; Fiber: 9g; Fat: 9g

MACROS: 30% Protein; 25% Fat; 45% Carbohydrates

Chocolate Granola

Homemade granola is one of the best things to make for topping smoothie bowls, toting as a snack, or enjoying with a splash of milk. Chocolate adds an extra layer of flavor to the seeds and nuts. Add a cup of dark chocolate chips to the finished, cooled granola.

4 cups rolled oats

½ cup pumpkin seeds

½ cup slivered almonds

½ cup sunflower seeds

2 scoops chocolate protein powder

¼ teaspoon sea salt

½ cup maple syrup

¼ cup unsweetened cocoa powder

2 tablespoons melted coconut oil

1 teaspoon pure vanilla extract

1. Preheat the oven to 325°F. Line a sheet pan with parchment paper.

2. In a medium bowl, combine the oats, pumpkin seeds, almonds, sunflower seeds, protein powder, and salt until well mixed.

3. In a small bowl, whisk together the maple syrup, cocoa powder, oil, and vanilla until blended.

4. Add the maple mixture to the oat mixture, and toss until all the ingredients are coated.

5. Spread the granola out on the prepared sheet pan.

6. Transfer the sheet pan to the oven, and bake, tossing several times, for about 30 minutes, or until the granola is lightly browned and crunchy. Remove from the oven. Let cool on the sheet pan. Break into large pieces, and refrigerate in a sealed container for up to 2 weeks.

FAT-LOSS TIP: Reduce the portion to ½ cup, or omit one of the nuts or seeds to drop the fat grams.

PER SERVING (~¾ CUP): Calories: 405; Protein: 19g; Total carbohydrates: 49g; Fiber: 8g; Fat: 17g

MACROS: 20% Protein; 32% Fat; 48% Carbohydrates

Peanut Butter and Strawberry Overnight Oats

PREP TIME: 10 minutes, plus overnight to soak | Serves 3 | **MUSCLE GAIN**

Overnight oats are not a new, trendy creation; this dish was enjoyed as muesli in European countries for centuries. Soaking rolled oats in milk and yogurt creates a soft, satisfying texture similar to a cooked dish but without the effort and time of cooking. If fresh strawberries aren't available, frozen will work well, or even try a tablespoon of strawberry preserves.

2 cups rolled oats

2 scoops vanilla or plain protein powder (vegan or unsweetened whey)

2 cups unsweetened almond milk

¾ cup plain Greek yogurt

¼ cup peanut butter

1 teaspoon pure vanilla extract

1½ cups sliced strawberries

1. Evenly divide the oats, protein powder, almond milk, yogurt, peanut butter, and vanilla between 3 canning jars or containers. Stir to combine well.

2. Top each with ½ cup of sliced strawberries, seal, and refrigerate overnight or up to 4 days.

FAT-LOSS TIP: Omit the peanut butter, and add sliced banana to reduce the calories and fat in this tasty recipe.

PER SERVING: Calories: 581; Protein: 36g; Total carbohydrates: 65g; Fiber: 12g; Fat: 20g

MACROS: 25% Protein; 27% Fat; 48% Carbohydrates

Lemon-Blueberry Baked Oatmeal Cups

PREP TIME: 10 minutes, plus 10 minutes to stand | COOK TIME: 25 minutes
Serves 6 | **FAT LOSS**

This recipe makes hearty muffins, but baked oatmeal has a cake-like texture, so it can be cut into convenient grab-and-go squares if you prefer. It can be enjoyed cold or warm, so it is ideal for meal prep. This is a vegan recipe, but whey-based protein powder and regular milk can be used instead.

Nonstick cooking spray, for coating the muffin tin

2 cups unsweetened almond milk

½ cup maple syrup

Grated zest and juice of 1 lemon

2 tablespoons ground flaxseed

2 teaspoons pure vanilla extract

4 cups rolled oats

2 scoops plain vegan protein powder

1 teaspoon baking powder

½ teaspoon ground cinnamon

½ teaspoon salt

1½ cups blueberries

1. Preheat the oven to 375°F. Spray a 12-cup muffin tin with nonstick cooking spray.

2. In a large bowl, whisk together the almond milk, maple syrup, lemon zest, lemon juice, flaxseed, and vanilla until blended.

3. Add the oats, protein powder, baking powder, cinnamon, and salt. Stir to combine.

4. Fold in the blueberries, and let the mixture stand for 10 minutes.

5. Divide the oatmeal mixture evenly between the prepared muffin cups.

6. Transfer the muffin tin to the oven, and bake for 20 to 22 minutes, or until the oatmeal has cooked through. Remove from the oven. Let the oatmeal cups cool in the muffin tin until cooled and completely set. Refrigerate any leftovers in a sealed container for up to 4 days or freeze for up to 1 month.

PER SERVING (2 MUFFINS): Calories: 400; Protein: 17g; Total carbohydrates: 68g; Fiber: 8g; Fat: 7g

MACROS: 20% Protein; 15% Fat; 65% Carbohydrates

Zucchini-Banana Muffins

PREP TIME: 10 minutes | **COOK TIME:** 30 minutes | Serves 6 | **FAT LOSS**

Zucchini is a popular ingredient for muffins because of its mild taste and the fact that it often seems to pile up in the garden in an alarming amount. This recipe is a fabulous way to use up the excess. These are the perfect choice for a grab-and-go breakfast, and the hearty oat and flaxseed base will keep you satisfied for hours.

1 cup oat flour

1 cup rolled oats

½ cup ground flaxseed

1 scoop plain protein powder

1 tablespoon baking powder

1 teaspoon ground cinnamon

½ teaspoon sea salt

⅔ cup plain Greek yogurt

½ cup maple syrup

½ cup banana, peeled and mashed

1 large egg

1 teaspoon pure vanilla extract

1½ cups finely shredded zucchini

1. Preheat the oven to 350°F. Line a 12-cup standard muffin tin with paper muffin cups.

2. In a large bowl, combine the oat flour, oats, flaxseed, protein powder, baking powder, cinnamon, and salt.

3. In a medium bowl, whisk together the yogurt, maple syrup, banana, egg, and vanilla until well combined.

4. Add the wet ingredients to the dry ingredients, and stir until just combined.

5. Stir in the zucchini.

6. Spoon the batter into the prepared muffin cups.

7. Transfer the muffin tin to the oven, and bake for 25 to 30 minutes, or until the muffins have browned on top and a toothpick inserted into the center of a muffin comes out clean. Remove from the oven. Serve. Refrigerate any leftovers in a sealed container for 5 days or freeze for up to 1 month.

MUSCLE-GAIN TIP: Increase the portion from 2 muffins to 3 muffins, and serve each muffin with a tablespoon of nut butter.

PER SERVING (2 MUFFINS): Calories: 298; Protein: 12g; Total carbohydrates: 47g; Fiber: 6g; Fat: 8g

MACROS: 20% Protein; 20% Fat; 60% Carbohydrates

Egg-Topped Sweet Potato Toast

PREP TIME: 10 minutes | COOK TIME: 5 minutes | Serves 1 | **FAT LOSS**

Place sweet potato in the toaster for a slightly crispy, browned slice without the mess or fuss. This dish uses those tasty slices as the base of this open-faced breakfast sandwich. Try fried eggs if runny yolks are your preference.

1 large sweet potato, cut into ¼-inch slices

Nonstick cooking spray, for coating the skillet

2 large eggs

2 large egg whites

1 cup chopped baby spinach

Sea salt

Freshly ground black pepper

1 scallion, green and white parts, chopped

1. Working in batches, toast the sweet potato slices in a toaster or toaster oven until lightly browned and tender, flipping them if needed.

2. While toasting the sweet potato, heat a large skillet over medium heat, and spray generously with cooking spray.

3. In a small bowl, whisk together the eggs, egg whites, and spinach. Season with salt and pepper.

4. Pour the egg mixture into the skillet, and scramble for about 5 minutes, or until just cooked through but still moist. Remove from the heat.

5. Top the sweet potato slices with the eggs and scallion.

MUSCLE-GAIN TIP: Add 2 or 3 slices of Canadian bacon or lean turkey bacon to the meal. This will add 65 calories, 12 grams of protein, and 1 gram of fat.

PER SERVING: Calories: 332; Protein: 24g; Total carbohydrates: 38g; Fiber: 6g; Fat: 10g

MACROS: 30% Protein; 25% Fat; 45% Carbohydrates

Breakfast Burritos

PREP TIME: 15 minutes | COOK TIME: 5 minutes | Serves 3 | **MUSCLE GAIN**

Stuff these burritos with scrambled tofu or eggs, depending on your preference. If more spice is desired, add chili powder to the tofu, or use hot salsa. If eating them right from the freezer, microwave at 30-second intervals until warmed through.

6 (8-inch) whole wheat tortillas

2 servings Easy Tofu Scramble (page 43)

1 cup fresh or frozen corn kernels

½ cup salsa

⅓ cup shredded cheddar cheese

1 ripe avocado, pitted, peeled, and chopped

1. Put the tortillas on a work surface, and evenly divide the tofu scramble, corn, salsa, cheese, and avocado between them.

2. Fold the sides of the tortilla over the filling, and roll up from the unfolded side to form a tight sealed package. Serve by microwaving each for 1 minute; or tuck individually into sealable plastic bags, and store in the refrigerator for up to 4 days or freeze for up to 1 month.

FAT-LOSS TIP: Instead of tortillas, scoop the filling and toppings into crunchy lettuce leaves. This will drop the calories by about 250, fat by 8 grams, and carbohydrates by 37 grams.

PER SERVING (2 BURRITOS): Calories: 684; Protein: 41g; Total carbohydrates: 67g; Fiber: 19g; Fat: 28g

MACROS: 25% Protein; 33% Fat; 42% Carbohydrates

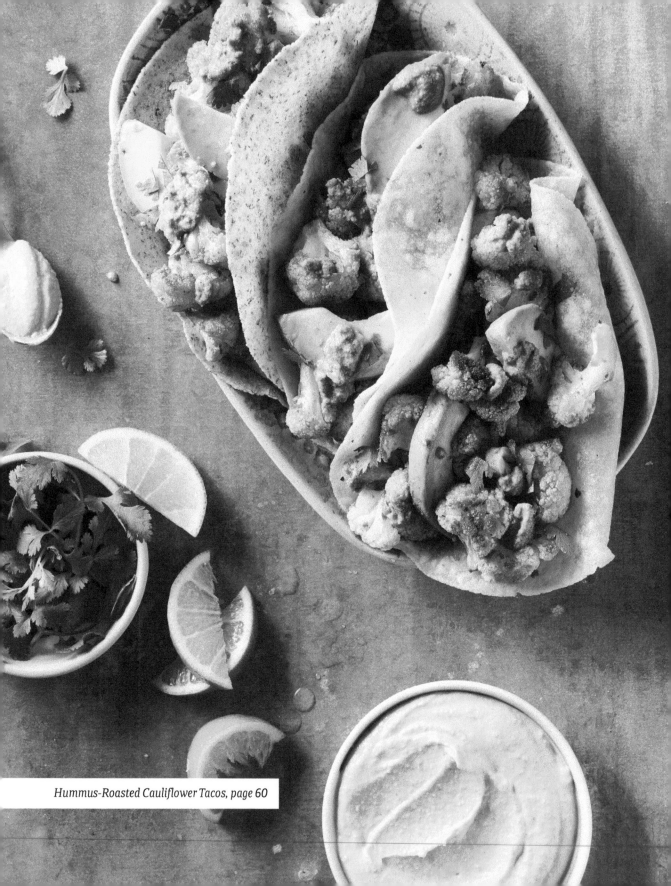

Hummus-Roasted Cauliflower Tacos, page 60

CHAPTER 4

PLANT-BASED MEALS

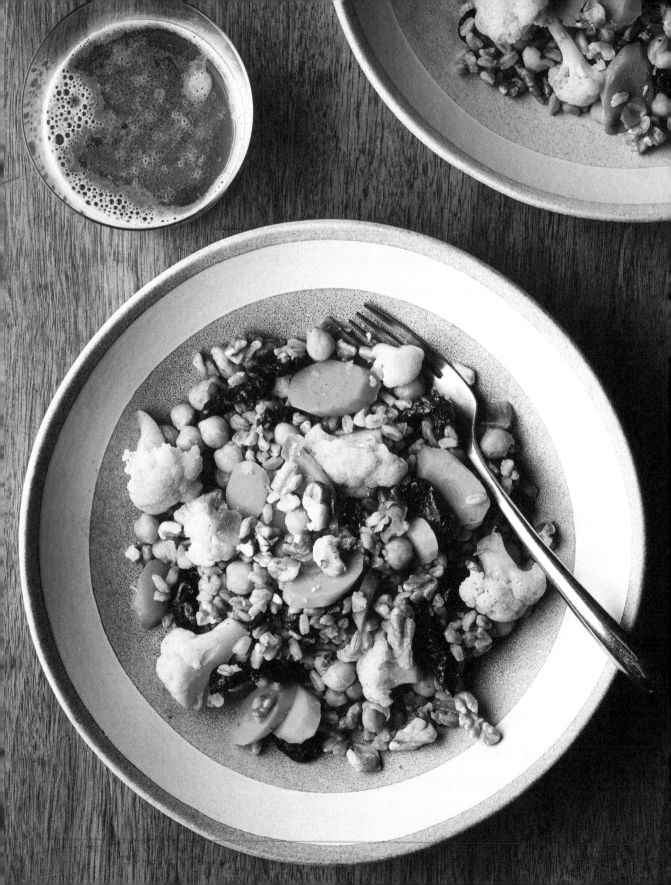

Moroccan-Inspired Seitan and Chickpeas

PREP TIME: 15 minutes | COOK TIME: 20 minutes | Serves 4 | FAT LOSS

North African food is resplendent with spices, dried fruit, nuts, and many protein-packed legumes and grains. If prunes aren't desired, try chopped dried apricots or fresh pomegranate arils.

1 small cauliflower, cut into small florets

3 carrots, cut into coins

1 (15-ounce) can chickpeas, drained and rinsed

1 (8-ounce) block seitan, cut into ½-inch chunks

1 small red onion, chopped

1 teaspoon minced garlic

1 tablespoon olive oil

1 teaspoon ground cumin

¼ teaspoon ground cinnamon

Sea salt

Freshly ground black pepper

½ cup pearled farro

1 cup water

½ cup chopped prunes

¼ cup chopped walnuts

1. Preheat the oven to 375°F. Line a sheet pan with parchment paper.

2. Spread the cauliflower, carrots, chickpeas, seitan, onion, and garlic out evenly on the prepared sheet pan. Drizzle with the oil, and season with the cumin, cinnamon, salt, and pepper. Toss to coat.

3. Transfer the sheet pan to the oven, and roast, tossing several times, for about 20 minutes, or until the vegetables are tender. Remove from the oven.

4. While the vegetables are roasting, in a medium saucepan, combine the farro and water. Bring to a boil over medium heat.

5. Reduce the heat to low. Cover the saucepan, and simmer for 12 to 15 minutes, or until the liquid has been absorbed. Remove from the heat. Let stand while the vegetables roast.

6. In a serving bowl, combine the roasted vegetables, farro, prunes, and walnuts. Toss until well mixed. Serve. Refrigerate any leftovers in sealed containers for up to 5 days or freeze for up to 1 month.

MUSCLE-GAIN TIP: Add a fried egg on top of each portion.

PER SERVING: Calories: 406; Protein: 25g; Total carbohydrates: 52g; Fiber: 12g; Fat: 11g

MACROS: 25% Protein; 25% Fat; 50% Carbohydrates

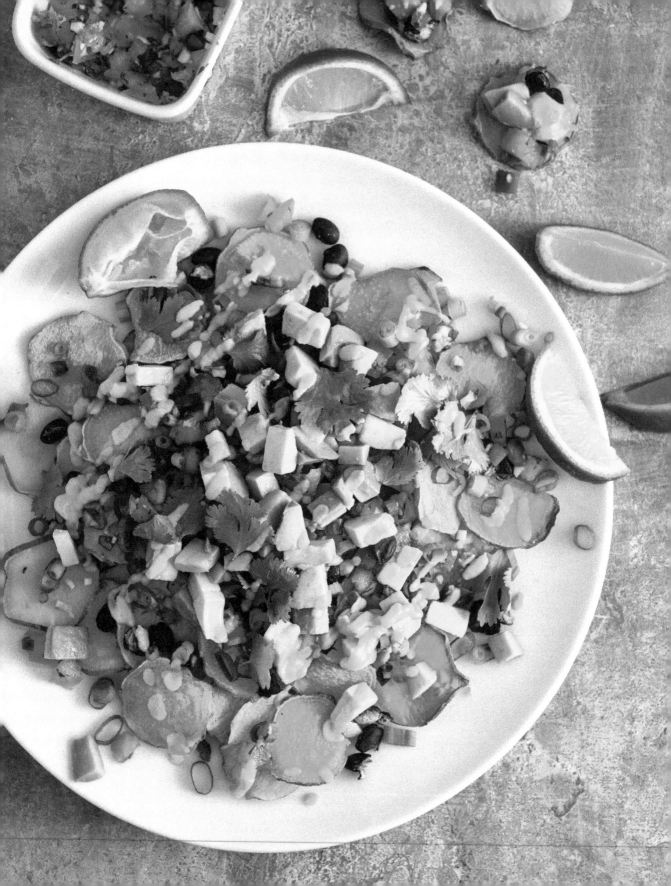

Sweet Potato Nachos

PREP TIME: 15 minutes | COOK TIME: 30 minutes | Serves 2 | **FAT LOSS**

Sweet potatoes provide a crispy, slightly sweet base for all the delicious toppings that make nachos one of many restaurants' most popular menu items. Any root vegetable works here, including beets, carrots, and parsnips. For extra-crispy sweet potato chips, soak the slices in cold water for 30 minutes, and pat them completely dry before baking them.

2 medium sweet potatoes, washed and cut into ¼-inch rounds

½ tablespoon olive oil

Sea salt

Freshly ground black pepper

1 tomato, chopped

¼ small onion, chopped

¼ jalapeño, chopped

¼ cup chopped fresh cilantro

Juice of 1 lime, divided

¼ cup plain Greek yogurt

1 tablespoon nutritional yeast

½ teaspoon ground cumin

Splash hot sauce

½ (15-ounce) can black beans, drained, rinsed, and patted dry

1 scallion, green part only, chopped

¼ large ripe avocado, pitted, peeled, and chopped

1. Preheat the oven to 400°F. Line a sheet pan with parchment paper.

2. Spread the sweet potato slices out on the prepared sheet pan. Toss with the oil. Season with salt and pepper.

3. Transfer the sheet pan to the oven, and bake, tossing several times, for 30 minutes, or until the sweet potatoes are very crispy and golden. Remove from the oven. Transfer to a serving platter.

4. While the sweet potatoes are baking, to make the tomato salsa, in a small bowl, combine the tomato, onion, jalapeño, cilantro, and juice of ½ lime until well mixed.

5. To make the yogurt sauce, in a small bowl, stir together the yogurt, nutritional yeast, cumin, hot sauce, and juice of the remaining ½ lime until smooth.

6. Top the sweet potatoes with the beans, tomato salsa, scallion, and avocado.

7. Drizzle with the yogurt sauce, and serve.

MUSCLE-GAIN TIP: Add 1 cup shredded cheddar cheese to increase the calories by 115, protein by 8 grams, and fat by 9 grams.

PER SERVING: Calories: 300; Protein: 15g; Total carbohydrates: 42g; Fiber: 12g; Fat: 8g

MACROS: 20% Protein; 25% Fat; 55% Carbohydrates

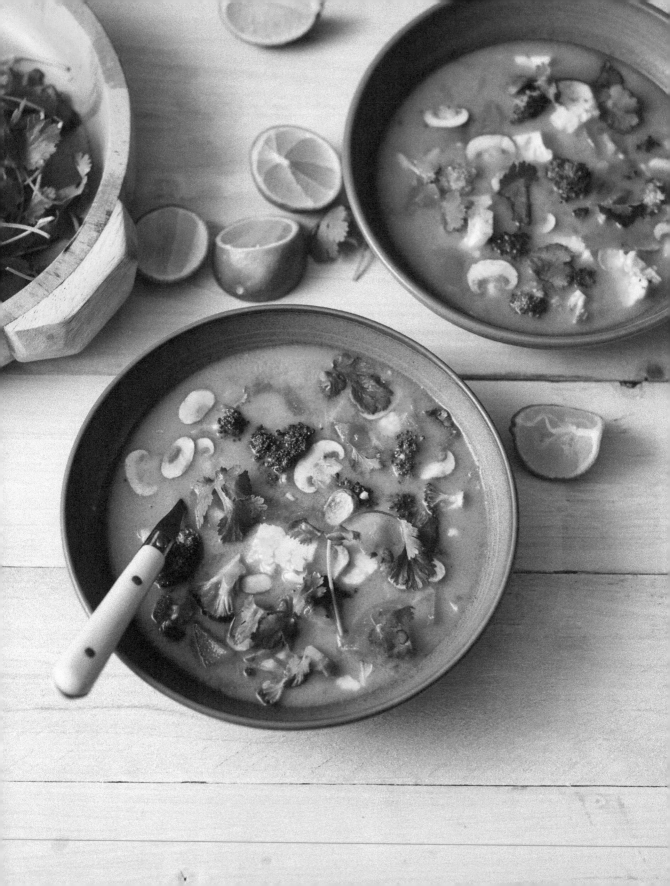

Vegetarian Tom Yum Soup

PREP TIME: 10 minutes | **COOK TIME:** 25 minutes | Serves 2 | **FAT LOSS**

This Thai soup is often served with chopped shrimp, but this creation is just as delicious. The hot and sour taste, tender-crisp vegetables, and flavor-packed tofu chunks combine in one balanced bowl. It is best made fresh but can also be enjoyed cold as a grab-and-go lunch.

6 cups low-sodium vegetable broth, divided

1 onion, chopped

1 small red chile pepper, chopped

1 tablespoon grated fresh ginger

1 tablespoon minced garlic

1½ cups thinly sliced mushrooms

2 tomatoes, chopped

½ (14-ounce) block extra-firm tofu, pressed and cut into ½-inch chunks

Juice of 1 lime

2 tablespoons curry paste

2 teaspoons coconut aminos

2 cups small broccoli florets

½ cup plain Greek yogurt

2 tablespoons chopped fresh cilantro

1. In a large stockpot, heat ¼ cup of broth over medium-high heat.

2. Add the onion, chile pepper, ginger, and garlic. Cook for about 3 minutes, or until softened.

3. Add the mushrooms, and sauté for 5 minutes.

4. Add the remaining 5¾ cups of broth, the tomatoes, tofu, lime juice, curry paste, and coconut aminos. Bring to a boil.

5. Reduce the heat to low. Simmer for 10 minutes to mellow the flavors.

6. Add the broccoli, and simmer for 2 minutes. Remove from the heat.

7. Whisk in the yogurt.

8. Serve the soup topped with the cilantro.

MUSCLE-GAIN TIP: Substitute 1 cup light coconut milk for the vegetable broth to create a creamy version of this soup. This will boost the calories, supplying lots of energy for a workout.

PER SERVING: Calories: 259; Protein: 21g; Total carbohydrates: 33g; Fiber: 10g; Fat: 9g

MACROS: 27% Protein; 27% Fat; 46% Carbohydrates

Hummus-Roasted Cauliflower Tacos

PREP TIME: 15 minutes | COOK TIME: 25 minutes | Serves 4 | **MUSCLE GAIN**

Cauliflower is incredibly versatile; it soaks up any added flavor and combines well with most ingredients. This cruciferous vegetable is not only delicious but also supports fat loss.

1 medium head cauliflower, cut into florets

2 teaspoons olive oil

1 cup store-bought hummus

Sea salt

8 (6-inch) high-protein whole wheat tortillas

¼ cup store-bought or homemade salsa verde

½ ripe avocado, pitted, peeled, and chopped

2 tablespoons chopped fresh cilantro

1 lime, cut into 6 wedges

1. Preheat the oven to 375°F. Line a sheet pan with parchment paper. Spread the cauliflower out on the prepared sheet pan. Toss with the oil.

2. Transfer the sheet pan to the oven, and roast, tossing halfway through, for about 10 minutes, or until the cauliflower is tender-crisp. Remove from the oven, leaving the oven on.

3. Toss the roasted florets with the hummus and salt until coated. Return the sheet pan to the oven, and roast for 10 to 15 minutes, or until the florets are crispy and golden brown. Remove from the oven.

4. Divide the florets between the tortillas and top with the salsa verde, avocado, and cilantro.

5. Serve the tacos with the lime wedges. Store the roasted cauliflower, salsa, and tortillas in separate containers. Toss the avocado with lime juice to prevent oxidation, then store in a small, sealed container.

FAT-LOSS TIP: Omit the hummus, and toss the cauliflower in ½ teaspoon paprika, ½ teaspoon cumin, and a pinch cayenne to cut the calories by 99. The macros will still be close to the original recipe.

PER SERVING: Calories: 437; Protein: 25g; Total carbohydrates: 55g; Fiber: 24g; Fat: 13g
MACROS: 24% Protein; 26% Fat; 50% Carbohydrates

Lentil Curry

PREP TIME: 10 minutes, plus 10 minutes to stand | COOK TIME: 25 minutes

Serves 4 | FAT LOSS

Curry is often a staple menu item in vegetarian-themed restaurants because it is incredibly versatile and delicious. Curry powder is not a single spice but rather a blend containing more than 30 herbs and spices. If heat is desired, try using hot curry powder or paste instead of mild.

2 teaspoons avocado oil

1 onion, chopped

1 tablespoon minced garlic

1 tablespoon curry powder

1 teaspoon ground cumin

2 cups low-sodium vegetable broth

2 (15-ounce) cans no-salt-added lentils, drained and rinsed

1 (15-ounce) can low-sodium crushed tomatoes

2 ounces seitan, crumbled

2 carrots, cut into ½-inch chunks

1 sweet potato, peeled and cut into ½-inch chunks

2 cups chopped kale

1. In a large stockpot, heat the oil over medium-high heat.

2. Add the onion, garlic, curry powder, and cumin. Sauté for about 3 minutes, or until the onion has softened.

3. Add the broth, lentils, tomatoes, seitan, carrots, and sweet potato. Bring to a boil.

4. Reduce the heat to low. Cover the pot, and simmer for about 15 minutes, or until the vegetables are tender and the liquid has reduced.

5. Add the kale. Remove from the heat. Let the curry stand for 10 minutes to wilt the greens. Serve. Refrigerate any leftovers in sealed containers for up to 5 days or freeze for up to 1 month.

FAT-LOSS TIP: Serve this curry over ½ cup brown rice or quinoa to add energy-boosting complex carbohydrates.

PER SERVING: Calories: 423; Protein: 29g; Total carbohydrates: 52g; Fiber: 17g; Fat: 11g

MACROS: 26% Protein; 24% Fat; 50% Carbohydrates

Smashed Avocado-Chickpea Toast

PREP TIME: 15 minutes | Serves 2 | **MUSCLE GAIN**

Avocado toast is a simple choice when something fast but rich with healthy fat and protein is needed. Adding chickpeas and cumin elevates this trendy dish, and the baby spinach adds iron. To save more time, use hummus in place of the chickpeas.

1 (14-ounce) can no-salt-added chickpeas, drained and rinsed

½ teaspoon ground cumin

Sea salt

4 toasted whole-grain bread slices

½ ripe avocado, pitted, peeled, and thinly sliced

1 cup baby spinach

1. In a medium bowl, combine the chickpeas and cumin. Season with salt. Using a fork, mash until the mixture is a thick paste.

2. Divide the mashed chickpeas between the toast slices, spreading evenly.

3. Top with the avocado and spinach. Serve open-faced.

FAT-LOSS TIP: Try a dense rye bread instead of regular bread to cut the calories by nearly 100 without dropping the protein significantly.

PER SERVING (2 SLICES): Calories: 485; Protein: 26g; Total carbohydrates: 66g; Fiber: 4g; Fat: 13g

MACROS: 23% Protein; 24% Fat; 53% Carbohydrates

Bean and Pumpkin Stew

PREP TIME: 15 minutes | COOK TIME: 25 minutes | Serves 3 | **FAT LOSS**

Stew does not need meat to be hearty and satisfying. Beans, starchy pumpkin, and edamame provide energy without adding too much fat. Most grocery stores carry frozen pumpkin if fresh pie pumpkins can't be found. In a pinch, substitute sweet potato or winter squash.

1 tablespoon olive oil

1 onion, chopped

3 celery stalks, chopped

1 tablespoon minced garlic

5 cups low-sodium vegetable broth

2 (15-ounce) cans no-salt-added great northern beans, drained and rinsed

4 cups fresh or frozen pumpkin, cut into ½-inch chunks

1 cup frozen edamame

2 teaspoons dried thyme

1 teaspoon dried oregano

2 cups baby spinach

¾ cup plain Greek yogurt

1. In a large stockpot, heat the oil over medium-high heat.

2. Add the onion, celery, and garlic. Sauté for about 3 minutes, or until softened.

3. Add the broth, beans, pumpkin, edamame, thyme, and oregano. Bring to a boil.

4. Reduce the heat to low. Cover the pot, and simmer for about 15 minutes, or until the vegetables are tender.

5. Add the spinach, and simmer for 2 minutes. Remove from the heat.

6. Serve the stew topped with yogurt.

MUSCLE-GAIN TIP: Tofu is an excellent addition to this hearty stew, or serve it with a slice of Ezekiel bread to boost protein and healthy fats.

PER SERVING: Calories: 409; Protein: 26g; Total carbohydrates: 61g; Fiber: 18g; Fat: 10g

MACROS: 24% Protein; 20% Fat; 56% Carbohydrates

Black Bean Veggie Burgers

PREP TIME: 10 minutes, plus 1 hour to chill | COOK TIME: 15 minutes
Serves 2 | **MUSCLE GAIN**

Who doesn't like a juicy burger smothered in toppings? These black bean patties make for a spectacular post-workout lunch or a tasty dinner after a long day. They contain 37 grams of protein, which is more than a 5-ounce beef burger, with 10 grams less fat. These burgers freeze well, so whip up a double batch, and keep the uncooked patties on hand for an easy meal later.

2 teaspoons olive oil, divided

½ onion, chopped

2 teaspoons minced garlic

2 cups no-salt-added black beans, drained and rinsed

1 carrot, shredded

1 large egg white

⅓ cup ground almonds

2 tablespoons chopped fresh parsley leaves

1 teaspoon ground cumin

Sea salt

Freshly ground black pepper

4 whole wheat buns, toasted

4 low-fat Swiss cheese slices

1. In a medium skillet, heat 1 teaspoon of oil over medium-high heat.

2. Add the onion and garlic. Sauté for about 3 minutes, or until softened. Remove from the heat. Transfer to a food processor.

3. Add the beans, carrot, egg white, almonds, parsley, and cumin. Season with salt and pepper. Pulse until the mixture holds together when pressed.

4. Divide the mixture into 8 portions, and form into patties. Cover, and refrigerate for 1 hour to firm up.

5. In a large skillet, heat the remaining 1 teaspoon of oil over medium heat.

6. Add all the patties, and cook, turning halfway through, for about 12 minutes, or until golden and heated through. Remove from the heat.

7. Serve the patties on buns with the cheese and favorite toppings.

FAT-LOSS TIP: Serve these filling patties on lettuce leaves instead of buns.

PER SERVING: Calories: 480; Protein: 37g; Total carbohydrates: 54g; Fiber: 20g; Fat: 14g

MACROS: 28% Protein; 25% Fat; 47% Carbohydrates

Green Spring Pasta

PREP TIME: 10 minutes | COOK TIME: 10 minutes | Serves 2 | **MUSCLE GAIN**

Primavera pasta usually features an array of colorful vegetables, but this complete palette of greens is very pleasing to the eye and taste buds. Green vegetables are usually the highest in protein and are an excellent source of nitrates linked to muscular performance.

4 ounces high-protein whole wheat penne or rotini pasta

2 tablespoons water or vegetable stock

1 zucchini, chopped

2 cups small broccoli florets

1 cup fresh or frozen peas

1 scallion, green and white parts, chopped

3 tablespoons basil pesto

2 cups shredded baby spinach

¼ cup shredded Parmesan cheese

1. Bring a large saucepan filled three-quarters full of water to a boil over high heat.

2. Add the pasta, and cook for about 10 minutes, or according to the package instructions. Remove from the heat. Drain.

3. While the pasta is cooking, in a large skillet, heat the 2 tablespoons of water over medium-high heat.

4. Add the zucchini, broccoli, peas, and scallion. Sauté for about 4 minutes, or until tender-crisp.

5. Add the pesto, and toss to coat.

6. Add the spinach. Sauté for about 2 minutes, or until wilted.

7. Add the cooked pasta and cheese. Toss to coat. Remove from the heat. Serve.

FAT-LOSS TIP: Increase the servings to 3 to cut the calories to 350 while keeping the macros the same.

PER SERVING: Calories: 526; Protein: 27g; Total carbohydrates: 64g; Fiber: 20g; Fat: 18g

MACROS: 21% Protein; 29% Fat; 50% Carbohydrates

Spicy Vegetarian Bulgur Chili

PREP TIME: 10 minutes | COOK TIME: 25 minutes | Serves 3 | FAT LOSS

Bulgur is a stellar choice for a quick meal. This ingredient is wheat kernels that are parboiled and cracked, so they take very little time to cook. If bulgur isn't available, try quinoa, farro, barley, or brown rice instead; just adjust the cooking time according to package instructions.

2 teaspoons olive oil

1 red bell pepper, cored and chopped

½ onion, chopped

2 teaspoons minced garlic

1 (15-ounce) no-salt-added diced tomatoes with their juices

1 (15-ounce) can no-salt-added white beans, drained and rinsed

1½ cups frozen edamame

1 cup no-salt-added vegetable broth

½ cup frozen or fresh corn kernels

½ cup bulgur

2 tablespoons chili powder

¼ teaspoon cayenne

½ cup shredded cheddar cheese

¼ cup sour cream

1 tablespoon chopped fresh cilantro

1. In a large stockpot, heat the oil over medium-high heat.

2. Add the bell pepper, onion, and garlic. Sauté for about 3 minutes, or until softened.

3. Add the tomatoes with their juices, the beans, edamame, broth, corn, bulgur, chili powder, and cayenne. Bring to a boil.

4. Reduce the heat to low. Partially cover, and simmer for about 15 minutes, or until the bulgur is tender and the chili is thick. Remove from the heat.

5. Serve the chili topped with the cheese, sour cream, and cilantro.

MUSCLE-GAIN TIP: Add seitan, tempeh, or tofu to boost the protein and calories.

PER SERVING: Calories: 411; Protein: 25g; Total carbohydrates: 58g; Fiber: 18g; Fat: 12g

MACROS: 23% Protein; 25% Fat; 52% Carbohydrates

Two-Bean Veggie Salad

PREP TIME: 15 minutes | Serves 2 | **MUSCLE GAIN**

This simple salad boasts 30 grams of protein per serving and 18 grams of fiber. Legumes and beans—like those in this delicious dish—are rich in the amino acids required for muscle gain. This is an excellent dish for a festive potluck dinner or family barbecue; just double it and go!

2 cups fresh or frozen edamame, thawed if frozen

1 (15-ounce) can no-salt-added kidney beans

1 English cucumber, chopped

1 cup halved cherry tomatoes

½ cup fresh or frozen corn

¼ cup feta cheese

¼ cup chopped fresh parsley

¼ cup store-bought low-fat balsamic dressing

1. In a large bowl, toss together the edamame, beans, cucumber, tomatoes, corn, cheese, and parsley until combined.

2. Add the dressing, and toss to coat. Serve, or refrigerate for up to 3 days.

FAT-LOSS TIP: Try this without the dressing, and use the juice of 1 lime or a splash of balsamic vinegar instead.

PER SERVING: Calories: 483; Protein: 30g; Total carbohydrates: 64g; Fiber: 18g; Fat: 14g

MACROS: 23% Protein; 25% Fat; 52% Carbohydrates

Mujadara

PREP TIME: 10 minutes | COOK TIME: 20 minutes | Serves 4 | **MUSCLE GAIN**

Mujadara has many variations—and spellings—across North Africa and the Middle East. This recipe is not traditional with the added tofu but stays true to the flavor profile. Any type of lentil works here, but green lentils have a firmer texture and are the classic choice.

¾ cup brown rice, soaked in 3 cups water overnight at room temperature

1½ cups water

2 teaspoons olive oil

2 onions, thinly sliced

1 (14-ounce) block extra-firm tofu, pressed (see page 43) and crumbled

2 tablespoons tahini

2 teaspoons minced garlic

1 teaspoon ground cumin

¼ teaspoon ground cinnamon

2 (15-ounce) cans no-salt-added lentils, drained and rinsed

Juice of ½ lemon

1. Drain the rice, and put in a large saucepan with the water. Bring to a boil over medium-high heat.

2. Reduce the heat to a simmer. Cover the saucepan, and simmer for about 15 minutes, or until the water has been completely absorbed and the rice is tender. Remove from the heat. Fluff with a fork.

3. While the rice is cooking, in a large skillet, heat the oil over medium-high heat.

4. Add the onions, and sauté for about 12 minutes, or until caramelized.

5. Add the tofu, tahini, garlic, cumin, and cinnamon. Sauté for 2 minutes.

6. Add the cooked rice and lentils, and stir. Remove from the heat.

7. Squeeze the lemon juice over the mujadara.

FAT-LOSS TIP: Omit the tofu, and increase the onions to 4 for a classic dish. This will reduce the number of calories and add complex carbohydrates and fiber.

PER SERVING: Calories: 498; Protein: 29g; Total carbohydrates: 64g; Fiber: 20g; Fat: 14g

MACROS: 24% Protein; 25% Fat; 51% Carbohydrates

Lentil Bolognese with Whole-Grain Spaghetti

PREP TIME: 10 minutes | COOK TIME: 20 minutes | Serves 2 | **MUSCLE GAIN**

How can a Bolognese sauce can be made with lentils instead of meat and still be called Bolognese? This sauce deserves the moniker because it is thick, rich, and has a texture very similar to the traditional sauce that inspired it. For increased decadence, stir in a splash of heavy cream for an authentic finish.

4 ounces protein-plus whole-grain spaghetti

2 teaspoons olive oil

2 cups chopped white mushrooms

½ onion, chopped

1 tablespoon minced garlic

1 (15-ounce) can no-salt-added lentils, drained and rinsed

1 (15-ounce) can no-salt-added crushed tomatoes

1 tablespoon dried oregano

2 teaspoons dried basil

¼ cup grated Parmesan cheese

1. Bring a large saucepan filled three-quarters full of water to a boil over high heat.

2. Add the spaghetti, and cook for about 10 minutes, or according to the package instructions. Remove from the heat. Drain.

3. While the spaghetti is cooking, to make the sauce, in a large skillet, heat the oil over medium-high heat.

4. Add the mushrooms, onion, and garlic. Sauté for about 5 minutes, or until softened.

5. Add the lentils, tomatoes, oregano, and basil. Bring to a simmer.

6. Reduce the heat to low. Simmer for about 10 minutes, or until heated through and the flavors mellow. Remove from the heat.

7. Top the cooked spaghetti with the sauce and cheese. Serve.

FAT-LOSS TIP: Increase the servings to 3 to decrease the calories to 397, and serve with a fresh green salad.

PER SERVING: Calories: 596; Protein: 32g; Total carbohydrates: 81g; Fiber: 4g; Fat: 16g

MACROS: 23% Protein; 24% Fat; 53% Carbohydrates

Mediterranean Tofu Quiche

PREP TIME: 15 minutes, plus 15 minutes to stand | COOK TIME: 30 minutes
Serves 3 | FAT LOSS

This low-fat, low-calorie recipe contains heaps of fiber-rich vegetables and a whopping 26 grams of protein. It does not freeze well but can be stored in the refrigerator for up to 5 days, making it great for meal prep.

Nonstick cooking spray, for coating the pie plate

4 tablespoons water, divided

1 cup sliced mushrooms

½ large onion, finely chopped

2 teaspoons minced garlic

2 cups small broccoli florets

1 cup asparagus, cut into 1½-inch pieces

½ cup shredded carrot

1 (14-ounce) block extra-firm tofu, pressed (see page 43)

1 cup great northern beans, drained and rinsed

2 tablespoons nutritional yeast

Sea salt

10 cherry tomatoes, halved

½ teaspoon chopped fresh thyme leaves

1. Preheat the oven to 375°F. Lightly spray a 9-inch pie plate with cooking spray.

2. In a large skillet, heat 2 tablespoons of water over medium-high heat. Add the mushrooms, onion, and garlic. Sauté for about 3 minutes, or until softened.

3. Add the broccoli, asparagus, and carrot. Sauté for 2 minutes. Remove from the heat.

4. While the vegetables are cooking, put the tofu, beans, and nutritional yeast in a blender. Blend at low speed, adding water by the tablespoon until the mixture is smooth, about 1 to 2 tablespoons. Turn off the blender. Season with salt. Pulse to combine.

5. Spread the cooked vegetables out on the pie plate and add the tomatoes and thyme. Pour the tofu mixture over the vegetables.

6. Transfer the pie plate to the oven, and bake for about 25 minutes, or until firm and a knife inserted into the center comes out hot. Remove from the oven. Let stand for 15 minutes before serving.

MUSCLE-GAIN TIP: Add ½ cup shredded Swiss or cheddar cheese to the tofu mixture.

PER SERVING: Calories: 278; Protein: 26g; Total carbohydrates: 32g; Fiber: 10g; Fat: 10g

MACROS: 29% Protein; 27% Fat; 44% Carbohydrates

Zucchini Ribbon Couscous Bowls

PREP TIME: 25 minutes | Serves 2 | **MUSCLE GAIN**

Couscous might look like a grain, but it is a pasta made with semolina or ground durum wheat. It is high in fiber and a good source of protein. In the same way a dish of pasta works for energy before a workout or playing sports, this dish is a quick no-cook choice that offers the same benefits and tons of taste.

FOR THE SAUCE

¼ cup plain soy milk

2 tablespoons tahini

Juice of 1 lime

FOR THE SALAD

½ cup whole wheat couscous

1 cup boiling water

2 zucchini, halved lengthwise and cut into long ribbons with a peeler

1 (15-ounce) can no-salt-added chickpeas, drained and rinsed

1 cup shredded red cabbage

½ cup halved cherry tomatoes

2 tablespoons roasted sunflower seeds

2 tablespoons hemp hearts

2 tablespoons chopped fresh cilantro

TO MAKE THE SAUCE

1. In a small bowl, whisk together the soy milk, tahini, and lime juice until smooth.

2. Thin the sauce with water until it can be drizzled, about 2 tablespoons.

TO MAKE THE SALAD

3. Put the couscous in a small bowl, and add the boiling water. Cover, and set aside for 10 minutes. Fluff with a fork.

4. In 2 serving bowls or containers, arrange the cooked couscous, zucchini ribbons, chickpeas, cabbage, tomatoes, sunflower seeds, hemp hearts, and cilantro.

5. Drizzle the salad with the sauce. Serve.

FAT-LOSS TIP: Reduce the chickpeas to 1 cup and omit the hemp hearts to drop the calories by 120 and keep the macros like the original recipe.

PER SERVING: Calories: 605; Protein: 30g; Total carbohydrates: 83g; Fiber: 18g; Fat: 17g

MACROS: 21% Protein; 24% Fat; 55% Carbohydrates

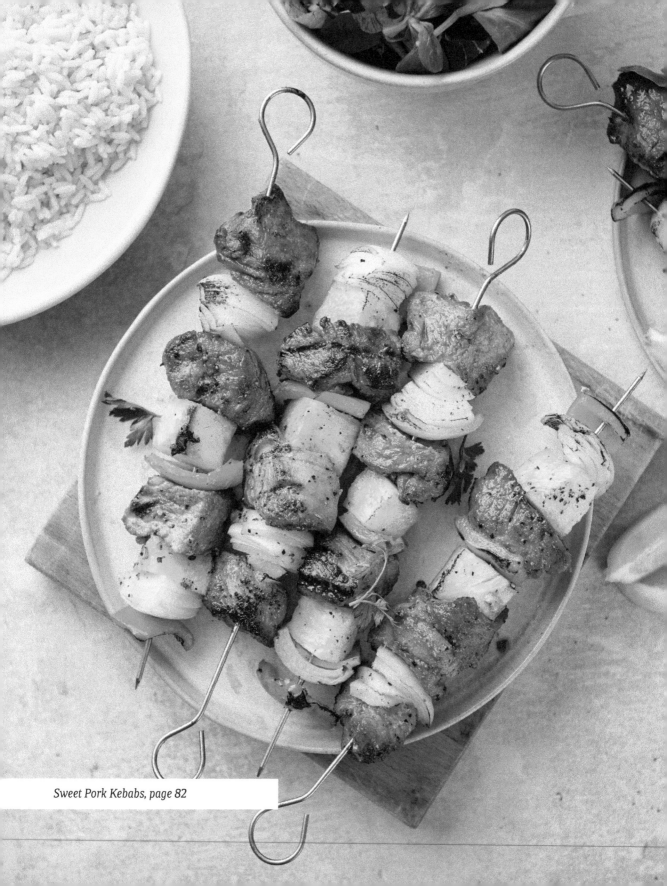

Sweet Pork Kebabs, page 82

FISH AND MEAT MEALS

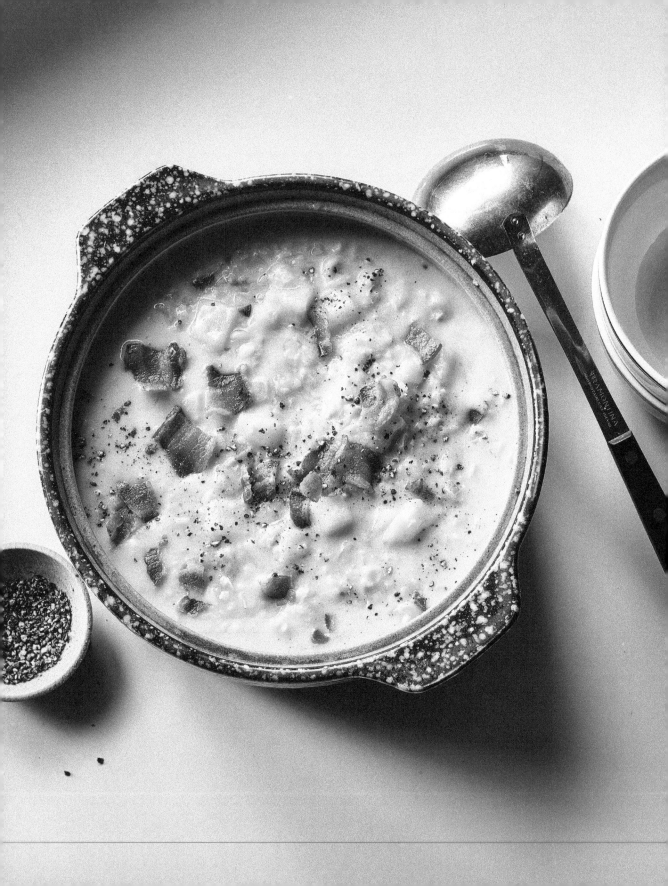

Creamy Corn Chowder

PREP TIME: 10 minutes | COOK TIME: 25 minutes | Serves 3 | **MUSCLE GAIN**

This recipe is a shortcut chowder made with creamed corn, creating a luscious texture without pureeing the soup in a blender. Skipping that step reduces the mess and the time spent making this dish. The bacon topping is a perfectly salty, crisp finish to the sweet corn.

2 teaspoons avocado oil

2 celery stalks, chopped

1 onion, chopped

2 teaspoons minced garlic

2 medium potatoes, peeled and cut into ½-inch chunks

2 (15-ounce) cans no-salt-added creamed corn

3 cups low-sodium vegetable broth

1 cup plain Greek yogurt

Sea salt

Freshly ground black pepper

8 cooked bacon slices, chopped

1. In a large saucepan, heat the oil over medium-high heat.

2. Add the celery, onion, and garlic. Sauté for about 5 minutes, or until softened.

3. Add the potatoes, creamed corn, and broth. Bring to a boil.

4. Reduce the heat to low. Simmer for about 15 minutes, or until the vegetables are tender. Remove from the heat.

5. Add the yogurt. Season with salt and pepper.

6. Serve the soup topped with the bacon.

FAT-LOSS TIP: Omit one of the potatoes to drop the calories; the consistency will be slightly thinner, but the flavor will be the same.

PER SERVING (~2½ CUPS): Calories: 520; Protein: 23g; Total carbohydrates: 79g; Fiber: 7g; Fat: 14g

MACROS: 18% Protein; 25% Fat; 57% Carbohydrates

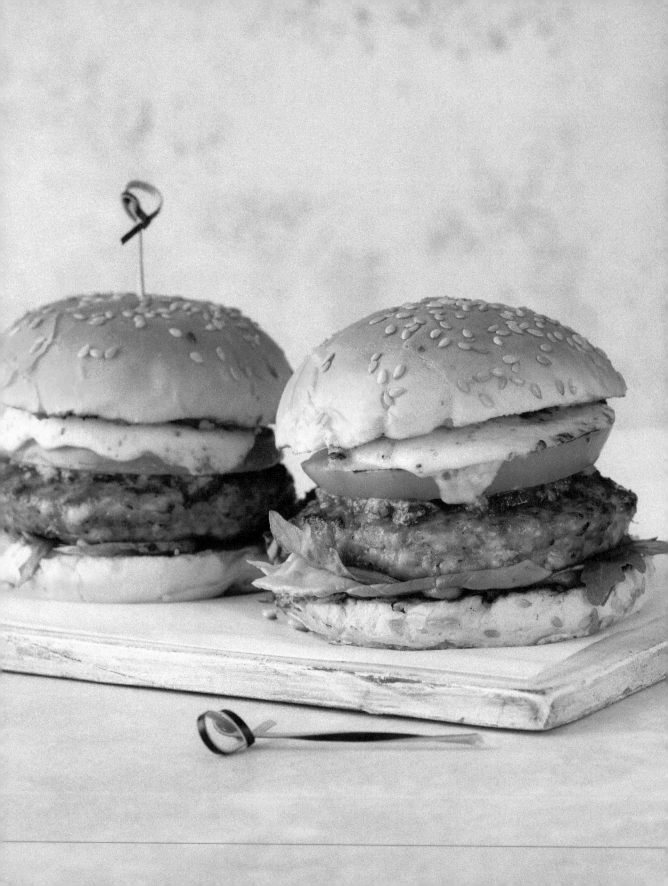

Caprese Turkey Burgers

PREP TIME: 10 minutes | COOK TIME: 20 minutes | Serves 4 | **FAT LOSS**

Turkey burgers are a delicious switch from standard beef burgers; they are lower in fat but still pack lots of protein. Top these with your favorite ingredients, such as bacon or sliced avocado. Swap out the turkey for chicken if that option is available.

1 pound extra-lean ground turkey

¼ cup bread crumbs

1 scallion, white part only, finely chopped

1 tablespoon chopped fresh parsley

1 teaspoon minced garlic

¼ teaspoon sea salt

¼ teaspoon paprika

⅛ teaspoon freshly ground black pepper

4 teaspoons store-bought basil pesto

1 large tomato, sliced

4 low-fat mozzarella cheese slices

4 lettuce leaves

4 whole wheat hamburger buns

1. Preheat the oven to 400°F. Line a sheet pan with parchment paper.

2. In a large bowl, combine the turkey, bread crumbs, scallion, parsley, garlic, salt, paprika, and pepper until evenly mixed.

3. Form the mixture into 4 equal patties, and place on the prepared sheet pan.

4. Transfer the sheet pan to the oven, and bake, turning halfway through, for about 15 minutes, or until the patties have cooked through. Remove from the oven, leaving the oven on.

5. Top each patty with the pesto, tomato, and cheese.

6. Return the sheet pan to the oven, and bake for about 2 minutes, or until the cheese melts. Remove from the oven.

7. Place the lettuce leaves on the bottom buns, then top with patties and remaining bun halves. Serve.

MUSCLE-GAIN TIP: If a calorie boost is needed for a workout, enjoy two of these burgers instead of one; the macros will stay the same.

PER SERVING (1 BURGER): Calories: 371; Protein: 39g; Total carbohydrates: 29g; Fiber: 2g; Fat: 10g

MACROS: 40% Protein; 27% Fat; 33% Carbohydrates

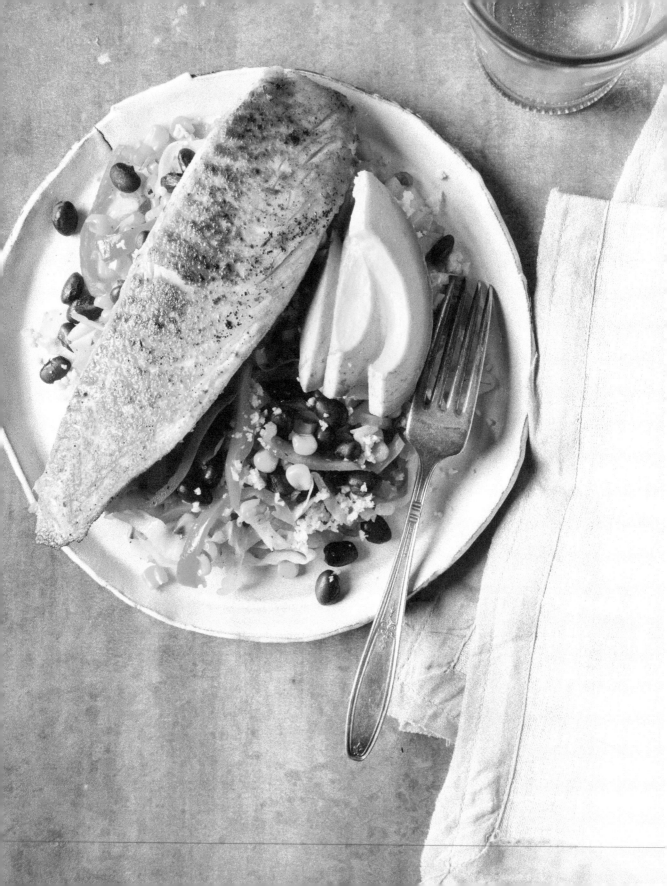

Trout Taco Bowls

PREP TIME: 15 minutes | COOK TIME: 10 minutes | Serves 2 | **FAT LOSS**

This dish is extremely attractive, perfect for a late supper outside on a warm evening. Trout is usually easy to find at the local grocery store, but haddock, halibut, or tilapia will suit the recipe as well. Flash-frozen fish are also an excellent option.

4 cups shredded cabbage

2 cups finely chopped cauliflower

1½ cups canned low-sodium corn

1 cup canned low-sodium black beans

1 red bell pepper, cored and thinly sliced

1 tablespoon olive oil, plus 1 teaspoon, divided

Juice of 1 lime

1 tablespoon granulated sugar

2 (4-ounce) skinless trout fillets

½ teaspoon ground cumin

½ teaspoon ground coriander

Sea salt

Freshly ground black pepper

1. In a large bowl, toss together the cabbage, cauliflower, corn, beans, and bell pepper until well mixed.

2. In a small bowl, whisk together 1 tablespoon of oil, the lime juice, and sugar. Pour over the vegetables, and toss to combine.

3. In a large skillet, heat the remaining 1 teaspoon of oil over medium-high heat.

4. Season the trout with the cumin, coriander, salt, and pepper.

5. Add the trout to the skillet and pan-sear, turning once, for about 10 minutes, or until golden and just cooked through. Remove from the heat.

6. Divide the vegetable mixture between 2 bowls, top with the trout, and serve.

MUSCLE-GAIN TIP: Tuck the fish and vegetable salad into a couple of corn or whole wheat tortillas instead of making a bowl.

PER SERVING (1 BOWL): Calories: 418; Protein: 28g; Total carbohydrates: 50g; Fiber: 15g; Fat: 14g

MACROS: 25% Protein; 30% Fat; 45% Carbohydrates

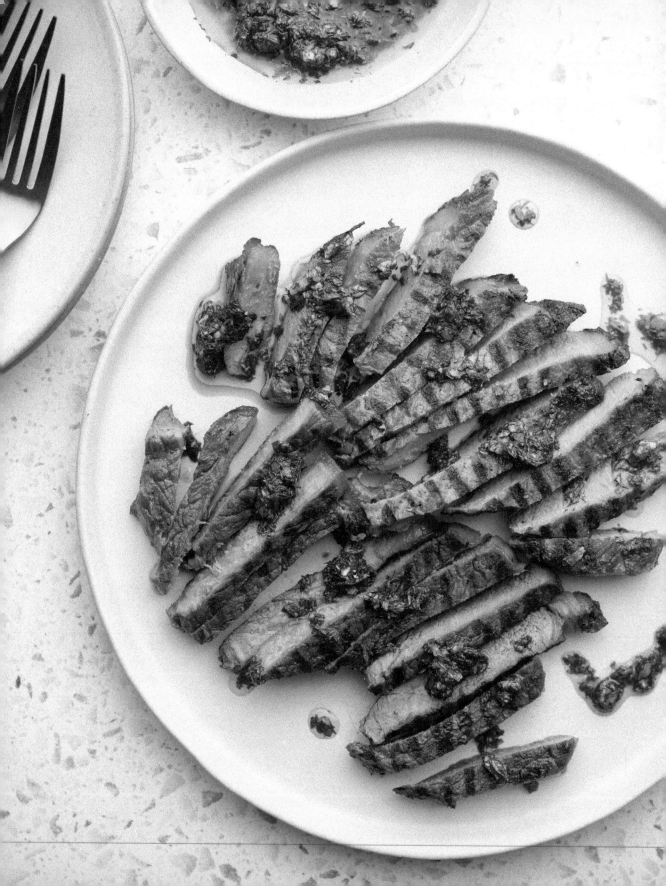

Sirloin with Chimichurri

PREP TIME: 10 minutes, plus 10 minutes to rest | COOK TIME: 15 minutes
Serves 2 | **MUSCLE GAIN**

Chimichurri is a green herb-based sauce used as a condiment and in cooking in South American cuisine. It packs a bit of heat, and the added vinegar and garlic create a bold flavor that stands up well to steak. Try a rib eye steak or tenderloin with this sauce.

FOR THE CHIMICHURRI

2 tablespoons olive oil

2 tablespoons chopped fresh parsley

½ tablespoon chopped fresh cilantro

½ tablespoon apple cider vinegar

1 teaspoon minced garlic

⅛ teaspoon sea salt

Pinch freshly ground black pepper

Pinch red pepper flakes

FOR THE STEAK

2 (6-ounce) sirloin strip steaks

Sea salt

Freshly ground black pepper

TO MAKE THE CHIMICHURRI

1. In a small bowl, stir together the oil, parsley, cilantro, vinegar, garlic, salt, pepper, and red pepper flakes.

TO MAKE THE STEAK

2. Bring the steaks to room temperature. Lightly season with salt and pepper.

3. Preheat the grill on high heat.

4. Put the steaks on the grill, and cook, turning halfway through, for 12 minutes for medium (140°F internal temperature), or until the desired doneness. (Or set the oven to broil, and broil the steaks on a sheet pan for the same time.) Remove from the heat. Let rest for 10 minutes.

5. Slice the steak thinly on a bias, and serve drizzled with the chimichurri.

FAT-LOSS TIP: Use a flank steak instead of sirloin to drop the fat grams. The lean cut is delicious and cooks in the same time.

PER SERVING (1 STEAK, 2 TABLESPOONS CHIMICHURRI):
Calories: 445; Protein: 35g; Total carbohydrates: 2g; Fiber: g; Fat: 31g

MACROS: 35% Protein; 62% Fat; 3% Carbohydrates

Sweet Pork Kebabs

PREP TIME: 10 minutes, plus at least 30 minutes to marinate
COOK TIME: 15 minutes | Serves 2 | **MUSCLE GAIN**

The marinade in this recipe is fabulous with other proteins like chicken and beef, and can be brushed on vegetables while grilling to create a lightly caramelized finish.

½ cup packed brown sugar

1 (15-ounce) can pineapple chunks in 100 percent fruit juice, with juice reserved

¼ cup low-sodium soy sauce

Juice of ½ lemon

2 teaspoons minced garlic

⅛ teaspoon sea salt

12 ounces boneless, thick-cut pork chops, cut into 1-inch chunks

1 onion, cut into eighths and then into 1-inch chunks

1 red bell pepper, cored and cut into 1-inch chunks

1. In a small bowl, whisk together the brown sugar, ¼ cup reserved pineapple juice, soy sauce, lemon juice, garlic, and salt to make a marinade. Reserve half of the marinade and set aside.

2. Add the pork chunks to the remaining half of the marinade. Refrigerate, and marinate for 30 minutes or up to 3 hours.

3. Preheat the oven to 450°F. Line a sheet pan with aluminum foil, and if a rack is available, place that on the sheet pan.

4. Alternating the ingredients, thread the pork, onion, bell pepper, and pineapple chunks onto skewers to make about 6 kebabs.

5. Place the kebabs on the prepared sheet pan. Brush with the reserved marinade. Transfer the sheet pan to the oven, and cook, turning several times, for about 12 minutes, or until the pork registers 145°F internal temperature and the vegetables have slightly charred on the edges. Brush the reserved marinade on the kebabs while turning. Remove from the oven. Serve.

FAT-LOSS TIP: Reduce the serving size to 2 kebabs. Serve with a huge green and vegetable salad.

PER SERVING (3 KEBABS): Calories: 556; Protein: 40g; Total carbohydrates: 72g; Fiber: 6g; Fat: 12g

MACROS: 30% Protein; 20% Fat; 50% Carbohydrates

Classic Chicken Noodle Soup

PREP TIME: 10 minutes | COOK TIME: 25 minutes | Serves 3 | FAT LOSS

There is something cozy about a steaming bowl of chicken noodle soup; it is the ideal light lunch when something healthy is desired. The noodles used here are skinny German-style noodles; very thin and about one and a half inches long. They can be found in most grocery and specialty stores in the pasta or soup section.

2 teaspoons olive oil

3 celery stalks, chopped

1 leek, white and light green parts, chopped and washed thoroughly

2 teaspoons minced garlic

6 cups low-sodium chicken broth

3 carrots, chopped

2 cups chopped chicken

2 cups soup egg noodles (thin)

Sea salt

Freshly ground black pepper

2 tablespoons chopped fresh parsley

1. In a large stockpot, heat the oil over medium-high heat.

2. Add the celery, leek, and garlic. Sauté for about 3 minutes, or until softened.

3. Add the broth, carrots, and chicken. Bring to a boil.

4. Reduce the heat to low. Simmer for 10 to 12 minutes, or until the carrots are tender.

5. Stir in the noodles, and simmer for 5 more minutes, or until softened. Remove from the heat. Season with salt and pepper.

6. Serve the soup topped with the parsley.

MUSCLE-GAIN TIP: Add a thick slice of whole-grain bread with a smear of butter for dipping.

PER SERVING (2½ CUPS): Calories: 297; Protein: 34g; Total carbohydrates: 42g; Fiber: 6g; Fat: 10g

MACROS: 32% Protein; 23% Fat; 45% Carbohydrates

Caldo Verde Soup

PREP TIME: 10 minutes | COOK TIME: 25 minutes | Serves 2 | **MUSCLE GAIN**

The broth in this traditional Portuguese soup is often flavored with ham hock. Turkey sausage stands in here, adding flavor and protein without the required time to simmer the hock. Pork sausage or a super spicy link can be used to create a unique version.

1 teaspoon olive oil

1 onion, chopped

1 tablespoon minced garlic

6 cups low-sodium chicken broth

2 potatoes, peeled and cut into ½-inch chunks

6 ounces spicy smoked turkey sausage, chopped

6 cups chopped kale

Sea salt

Freshly ground black pepper

1. In a large stockpot, heat the oil over medium-high heat.

2. Add the onion and garlic. Sauté for about 3 minutes, or until softened.

3. Add the broth and potatoes. Bring to a boil.

4. Reduce the heat to low. Simmer for about 14 minutes, or until the potatoes are tender. Remove from the heat. Transfer the soup to a blender. Puree, and return to the pot. (Or use an immersion blender.)

5. Add the sausage and kale. Simmer for about 3 minutes, or until the greens are tender. Remove from the heat. Season with salt and pepper. Serve.

FAT-LOSS TIP: Reduce the portion size and total calories by increasing the total servings to 3. This modification won't change the macros.

PER SERVING (3 CUPS): Calories: 500; Protein: 29g; Total carbohydrates: 65g; Fiber: 9g; Fat: 15g

MACROS: 24% Protein; 25% Fat; 51% Carbohydrates

Spinach, Chicken, and Lentil Salad

PREP TIME: 25 minutes | Serves 2 | **FAT LOSS**

Sometimes a simple but filling salad is what's needed at the end of a busy day, especially in warm summer months when no one wants to use a stove or grill. This dish is a full plate of vegetables, legumes, and chicken, so no one will be leaving the table feeling hungry.

8 cups baby spinach

1 English cucumber, chopped

3 cups green beans, trimmed and cut into 1-inch pieces

2 large tomatoes, chopped

2 or 3 thin slices red onion, separated into rings

5 or 6 tablespoons store-bought or homemade balsamic dressing

1½ cups chopped cooked chicken (store-bought rotisserie chicken or leftovers)

1 (15-ounce) can no-salt-added lentils, drained and rinsed

1. In a large bowl, toss together the spinach, cucumber, green beans, tomatoes, onion, and dressing.

2. Arrange the salad on 2 plates.

3. Top each salad with the chicken and lentils. Serve.

MUSCLE-GAIN TIP: Increase the amount of chicken, or add a couple slices of chopped bacon to the meal.

PER SERVING (1 SALAD): Calories: 410; Protein: 34g; Total carbohydrates: 43g; Fiber: 15g; Fat: 13g

MACROS: 31% Protein; 28% Fat; 41% Carbohydrates

Chicken, Spinach, and Pea Salad

PREP TIME: 25 minutes | Serves 2 | **FAT LOSS**

The combination of crisp, fresh vegetables, creamy dressing, chicken, crunchy pecans, and tart cranberries creates a salad packed with texture, flavor, and color. This salad is perfect for special company. Any dark leafy green works here, so try baby kale instead of spinach.

6 cups baby spinach

2 cups sliced white mushrooms

2 cups fresh peas

2 large tomatoes, chopped

2 thin slices red onion, separated into rings

¼ cup store-bought fat-free ranch dressing

1 cup chopped cooked chicken (store-bought rotisserie chicken or leftovers)

¼ cup chopped pecans

¼ cup dried cranberries

1. In a large bowl, toss together the spinach, mushrooms, peas, tomatoes, and onion with the dressing.

2. Evenly divide the greens between 2 plates.

3. Top each salad with the chicken, pecans, and cranberries. Serve.

MUSCLE-GAIN TIP: Swap out the fat-free dressing for regular to increase the calories and fat in the dish.

PER SERVING (1 SALAD): Calories: 471; Protein: 33g; Total carbohydrates: 57g; Fiber: 14g; Fat: 15g

MACROS: 25% Protein; 27% Fat; 48% Carbohydrates

Sheet Pan Shrimp Tacos

PREP TIME: 15 minutes | COOK TIME: 10 minutes | Serves 2 | **MUSCLE GAIN**

Shrimp is an ideal protein to make on a sheet pan because it cooks very quickly; this is excellent for this recipe because it means the vegetables retain their texture, too. The spices have some heat, so reduce or omit the chili powder if it's too hot. If leaving out the chili, add 1/4 teaspoon paprika to create the pretty color on the shrimp.

12 ounces (26⁄30 count per pound) shrimp, peeled, deveined, and tail off

1 red bell pepper, cored and thinly sliced

1 yellow bell pepper, cored and thinly sliced

½ red onion, thinly sliced

1 tablespoon olive oil

1 teaspoon chili powder

½ teaspoon garlic powder

½ teaspoon ground cumin

6 (6-inch) corn tortillas

½ cup store-bought or homemade salsa

2 tablespoons sour cream

Chopped fresh cilantro, for garnish

1. Preheat the oven to 400°F. Line a sheet pan with parchment paper.

2. Spread the shrimp, bell peppers, and onion out on the prepared sheet pan. Drizzle with the oil. Season with the chili powder, garlic powder, and cumin. Toss to coat, and spread everything out again.

3. Transfer the sheet pan to the oven, and bake for about 8 minutes, or until the shrimp have cooked through and the vegetables are tender.

4. Set the oven to broil. Broil for about 1 minute, or until the vegetables are lightly charred. Remove from the oven.

5. Evenly divide the shrimp and vegetables between the tortillas.

6. Top with the salsa, sour cream, and cilantro.

FAT-LOSS TIP: Replace the tortillas with lettuce leaves, and add baked tortilla strips as a crunchy topping.

PER SERVING (3 TACOS): Calories: 464; Protein: 31g; Total carbohydrates: 58g; Fiber: 9g; Fat: 14g

MACROS: 25% Protein; 25% Fat; 50% Carbohydrates

Simple Jambalaya

PREP TIME: 10 minutes | COOK TIME: 30 minutes | Serves 4 | FAT LOSS

Jambalaya is a Creole dish inspired by many different cuisines, like Spanish, French, and West African. To create a true Cajun version, omit the tomatoes. To save time, cook the rice ahead, and add it to the skillet along with the other ingredients after sautéing the vegetables. Then sauté until everything is heated through, and serve.

1 tablespoon olive oil

2 celery stalks, chopped

1 onion, chopped

1 tablespoon minced garlic

1 cup brown rice, soaked overnight at room temperature in 3 cups water and drained

2 cups low-sodium chicken broth

1 (15-ounce) can diced tomatoes with their juices

1 cup canned low-sodium red kidney beans, drained and rinsed

1 tablespoon Cajun or Creole seasoning mix

4 ounces (26/30 count per pound) shrimp, peeled, deveined, and chopped

2 cups chopped cooked chicken (store-bought rotisserie chicken or leftovers)

Freshly ground black pepper

1. In a large skillet, heat the oil over medium-high heat.

2. Add the celery, onion, and garlic. Sauté for about 3 minutes, or until softened.

3. Add the rice, broth, tomatoes with their juices, the beans, and seasoning mix. Bring to a boil.

4. Reduce the heat to low. Partially cover the skillet, and simmer for about 20 minutes, or until the rice is almost tender.

5. Add the shrimp and chicken. Cook for about 3 minutes, or until the shrimp is pink. Season with pepper. Serve.

MUSCLE-GAIN TIP: Increase the amount of shrimp and add a couple of links of sliced spicy sausage to create a classic jambalaya and increase the calories, fat, and protein.

PER SERVING (¼ RECIPE): Calories: 424; Protein: 34g; Total carbohydrates: 54g; Fiber: 8g; Fat: 9g

MACROS: 30% Protein; 18% Fat; 52% Carbohydrates

Sheet Pan Salmon with Mixed Vegetables

PREP TIME: 10 minutes | **COOK TIME:** 15 minutes | Serves 2 | **MUSCLE GAIN**

This meal looks delicious in the sheet pan with the spread of colorful vegetables and pink salmon fillets. Fish high in omega-3 fatty acids—like salmon—might help increase muscle gain, so fill up on this moist, delicious fish!

1 bunch broccoli, cut into small florets

¼ medium head cauliflower, cut into florets

2 parsnips, peeled and cut into ½-inch chunks

2 carrots, cut into ½-inch chunks

1 sweet potato, peeled and cut into ½-inch chunks

2 teaspoons olive oil

1 teaspoon ground cumin

Sea salt

Freshly ground black pepper

2 (6-ounce) skinless salmon fillets

2 tablespoons freshly squeezed lemon juice

½ teaspoon chopped fresh thyme leaves

1. Preheat the oven to 425°F. Line a sheet pan with parchment paper.

2. Spread the broccoli, cauliflower, parsnips, carrots, and sweet potato out on two-thirds of the prepared sheet pan. Drizzle with the oil. Season with the cumin, salt, and pepper. Toss to coat.

3. Place the salmon fillets on the remaining third of the sheet pan.

4. Drizzle the fillets with the lemon juice, and sprinkle with the thyme.

5. Transfer the sheet pan to the oven, and roast for about 15 minutes, or until the salmon has just cooked through and the vegetables are tender. Remove from the oven.

FAT-LOSS TIP: Omit the sweet potato; the parsnips are already starchy, so the meal will still be filling.

PER SERVING (1 FILLET, ½ THE VEGETABLES): Calories: 559; Protein: 40g; Total carbohydrates: 69g; Fiber: 20g; Fat: 14g

MACROS: 29% Protein; 24% Fat; 47% Carbohydrates

Angel-Hair Pasta with Tuna and Asparagus

PREP TIME: 10 minutes | COOK TIME: 15 minutes | Serves 3 | **FAT LOSS**

Good-quality canned fish is a stellar choice for many delicious recipes, even pasta with tender-crisp asparagus and lemon-herb sauce. Don't stir the pasta too much after adding the tuna; it should remain in chunks. This recipe is nice with chopped fresh dill as well.

6 ounces whole wheat angel-hair pasta

2 tablespoons olive oil

1 leek, white and light green parts, chopped and thoroughly washed

2 teaspoons minced garlic

1 large bunch asparagus, trimmed and cut into 2-inch pieces

Grated zest and juice of ½ lemon

2 (5-ounce) cans water-packed solid chunk tuna, drained

1 tablespoon chopped fresh parsley

Sea salt

Freshly ground black pepper

1. Bring a large saucepan filled three-quarters full of water to a boil over high heat.

2. Add the pasta, and cook for about 6 to 7 minutes, or according to the package instructions. Remove from the heat. Drain.

3. While the pasta is cooking, in a large skillet, heat the oil over medium-high heat.

4. Add the leek and garlic. Sauté for about 4 minutes, or until softened.

5. Add the asparagus, lemon zest, and lemon juice. Sauté for about 3 minutes, or until the asparagus is tender.

6. Add the tuna, and toss for about 4 minutes, or until heated through.

7. Add the cooked pasta and parsley. Toss. Season with salt and pepper. Serve. Refrigerate any leftovers for up to 3 days.

MUSCLE-GAIN TIP: Increase the tuna to 3 cans because this fish is high in omega-3 fatty acids and high-quality protein.

PER SERVING (⅓ RECIPE): Calories: 417; Protein: 29g; Total carbohydrates: 52g; Fiber: 7g; Fat: 12g

MACROS: 26% Protein; 25% Fat; 49% Carbohydrates

Salmon-Avocado Lettuce Wraps

PREP TIME: 20 minutes | Serves 3 | **FAT LOSS**

Mashed chickpeas have a creamy texture that replaces the traditional mayonnaise in this vegetable- and salmon-filled wrap. Tuck the filling into whole-grain tortillas for an easy grab-and-go meal. You can also use leftover cooked salmon from another meal instead of canned fish.

2 (5-ounce) cans water-packed boneless salmon

1 (15-ounce) can no-salt-added chickpeas, drained, rinsed, and mashed

2 carrots, shredded

2 celery stalks, chopped

2 tablespoons chopped red onion

Grated zest of ½ lime

¼ teaspoon minced garlic

1 ripe avocado, pitted, peeled, and diced

Sea salt

Freshly ground black pepper

6 large lettuce leaves

1. In a medium bowl, combine the salmon, chickpeas, carrots, celery, onion, lime zest, garlic, and avocado. Season with salt and pepper.

2. Scoop the salmon mixture into the lettuce leaves. Serve. Refrigerate the filling for up to 2 days.

MUSCLE-GAIN TIP: Bump the serving to 3 lettuce wraps to increase the calories to 646 per serving.

PER SERVING (2 LETTUCE WRAPS): Calories: 431; Protein: 40g; Total carbohydrates: 50g; Fiber: 15g; Fat: 9g

MACROS: 33% Protein; 20% Fat; 47% Carbohydrates

Bruschetta Chicken

PREP TIME: 10 minutes | **COOK TIME:** 20 minutes | Serves 2 | **FAT LOSS**

To balance the macros to suit the recommendations in this book, add complex carbohydrates to the meat with a side of grains or legumes. This recipe would be delicious served over brown rice, quinoa, or whole wheat couscous. Chicken is an excellent choice for weight loss because it is packed with protein.

FOR THE CHICKEN

8 ounces boneless, skinless chicken breasts, thinly sliced

1 teaspoon Italian seasoning

Sea salt

8 cups baby spinach

¼ cup low-sodium chicken broth

FOR THE BRUSCHETTA

4 large tomatoes, chopped

½ red onion, chopped

¼ cup chopped fresh basil leaves

1 teaspoon minced garlic

1 tablespoon balsamic vinegar

Sea salt

Freshly ground black pepper

¼ cup shredded Parmesan cheese

TO MAKE THE CHICKEN

1. Preheat the oven to 400°F. Line a sheet pan with parchment paper.

2. Season the chicken with the Italian seasoning and salt.

3. Spread the chicken out on half of the prepared sheet pan. Spread the spinach on the other half.

4. Drizzle the spinach with the broth. Season with salt.

5. Transfer the sheet pan to the oven, and bake, turning halfway through, for 15 minutes, or until the chicken has just cooked through and the spinach wilts. Remove from the oven, leaving the oven on.

TO MAKE THE BRUSCHETTA

6. While the chicken is cooking, in a small bowl, combine the tomatoes, onion, basil, garlic, and vinegar. Season with salt and pepper.

7. Spoon the bruschetta mixture over the cooked chicken.

8. Sprinkle with the cheese.

9. Transfer the wilted spinach to 2 plates.

10. Set the oven to broil.

11. Return the sheet pan to the oven. Broil for about 3 minutes, or until the cheese melts. Remove from the oven.

12. Serve the chicken and bruschetta mixture on the spinach.

MUSCLE-GAIN TIP: Toss the spinach, chicken, and bruschetta with pasta to add carbohydrates and calories to the meal.

PER SERVING (½ RECIPE): Calories: 303; Protein: 35g; Total carbohydrates: 25g; Fiber: 4g; Fat: 8g

MACROS: 40% Protein; 25% Fat; 35% Carbohydrates

Pork, Winter Squash, and Cranberry Sauté

PREP TIME: 10 minutes | COOK TIME: 30 minutes | Serves 2 | **MUSCLE GAIN**

This dish is like autumn in a skillet; maybe it is the tart cranberries and bright squash. Winter squash—like acorn and butternut—is high in fiber and carbohydrates and low on the glycemic index. This combination means it is a rich source of long-term energy for muscle recovery after exercise.

2 teaspoons olive oil

12 ounces extra-lean ground pork

4 cups diced (½-inch) winter squash

3 celery stalks, chopped

½ cup chopped onion

1 cup fresh cranberries

¼ cup maple syrup

½ teaspoon ground nutmeg

½ teaspoon dried thyme

Sea salt

Freshly ground black pepper

1. In a large skillet, heat the oil over medium-high heat.

2. Add the pork, and sauté for about 10 minutes, or until just cooked through.

3. Add the squash, celery, and onion. Sauté for about 10 minutes, or until softened.

4. Add the cranberries, maple syrup, nutmeg, and thyme. Sauté for about 10 minutes, or until the berries burst. Remove from the heat. Season with salt and pepper.

FAT-LOSS TIP: Cut the winter squash by 1 cup and the maple syrup by 1 tablespoon to reduce the calories. Bump the pork to 1 pound to increase protein and promote fat loss.

PER SERVING (½ RECIPE): Calories: 551; Protein: 40g; Total carbohydrates: 73g; Fiber: 10g; Fat: 14g

MACROS: 26% Protein; 24% Fat; 50% Carbohydrates

Mediterranean Pork Skillet

PREP TIME: 10 minutes | COOK TIME: 20 minutes | Serves 2 | **MUSCLE GAIN**

When thinking of Mediterranean food, many of the ingredients in this delicious dish will come to mind. Bell peppers, olives, garlic, artichoke hearts, and oregano combine with lean pork and fiber-packed bulgur for a spectacular meal. Look for artichoke hearts packed in water or light brine instead of oil for the best results.

1 tablespoon olive oil

8 ounces boneless center-cut pork chops, thinly sliced

2 bell peppers (red, orange, or yellow), cored and chopped

½ onion, chopped

2 teaspoons minced garlic

1 (28-ounce) can low-sodium diced tomatoes

1 cup canned quartered artichoke hearts

½ cup bulgur

¼ cup low-sodium chicken broth

¼ cup sliced kalamata olives

2 tablespoons chopped fresh oregano leaves

Pinch red pepper flakes

Sea salt

Freshly ground black pepper

1. In a large skillet, heat the oil over medium-high heat.

2. Add the pork, and sauté for about 7 minutes, or until no longer pink. Using a slotted spoon, transfer to a plate.

3. To the skillet, add the peppers, onion, and garlic. Sauté for about 4 minutes, or until softened.

4. Add the pork back to the skillet, and add the tomatoes, artichoke hearts, bulgur, broth, olives, oregano, and red pepper flakes.

5. Reduce the heat to medium-low. Cook for about 9 minutes, or until the bulgur is tender. Season with salt and pepper. Serve.

FAT-LOSS TIP: Increase the servings to 3 to reduce the calories without changing the macros.

PER SERVING (½ RECIPE): Calories: 525; Protein: 37g; Total carbohydrates: 63g; Fiber: 21g; Fat: 17g

MACROS: 27% Protein; 27% Fat; 46% Carbohydrates

Pork and Kale Pasta

PREP TIME: 10 minutes | COOK TIME: 15 minutes | Serves 3 | **MUSCLE GAIN**

This filling dish has few ingredients and tons of color and flavor. It is inspired by spaghetti aglio e olio, but pork is added here to increase the protein. If this is too spicy, omit the red pepper flakes.

8 ounces whole-grain penne pasta

8 ounces extra-lean ground pork

2 tablespoons salted butter

2 teaspoons minced garlic

8 cups shredded kale

⅛ teaspoon red pepper flakes

Sea salt

¼ cup grated Parmesan cheese

1. Bring a large saucepan filled three-quarters full of water to a boil over high heat.

2. Add the pasta, and cook for about 10 minutes, or according to the package instructions. Remove from the heat. Drain.

3. While the pasta is cooking, put the pork in a large skillet, and sauté over medium heat for about 6 minutes, or until cooked through. Using a slotted spoon, transfer to a plate.

4. Increase the heat to medium-high. In the same skillet, melt the butter.

5. Add the garlic, and sauté for about 3 minutes, or until softened.

6. Add the kale, and sauté for about 5 minutes, or until tender.

7. Add the red pepper flakes. Season with salt.

8. Add the cooked pasta, pork, and cheese. Toss. Remove from the heat. Serve.

FAT-LOSS TIP: Reduce the amount of pasta to 6 ounces, and use 12 ounces ground pork. This will decrease the calories while increasing the protein to 30 percent.

PER SERVING (⅓ RECIPE): Calories: 481; Protein: 31g; Total carbohydrates: 62g; Fiber: 8g; Fat: 14g

MACROS: 25% Protein; 25% Fat; 50% Carbohydrates

Beef Meat Loaf Muffins

PREP TIME: 10 minutes | COOK TIME: 35 minutes | Serves 4 | **FAT LOSS**

What could be more convenient than muffin-size meat loaves that can be frozen, eaten as is, or halved and tucked into whole wheat pitas? Beef is packed with protein, B vitamins, and creatine, which support weight loss and muscle gain. Try these with ground pork, lamb, chicken, or turkey to switch it up.

Nonstick cooking spray, for coating the muffin tin

8 ounces mushrooms

½ onion, coarsely chopped

1 large carrot, coarsely chopped

2 garlic cloves, peeled

2 teaspoons olive oil

1 pound extra-lean ground beef

½ cup bread crumbs

¼ cup milk

1 teaspoon chopped fresh thyme leaves

Sea salt

Freshly ground black pepper

½ cup ketchup

¼ cup packed brown sugar

1 tablespoon yellow mustard

1. Preheat the oven to 375°F. Spray a 12-cup muffin tin with cooking spray.

2. Put the mushrooms, onion, carrot, and garlic in a blender. Pulse until very finely chopped.

3. In a large skillet, heat the oil over medium-high heat.

4. Add the chopped vegetables, and sauté for about 4 minutes, or until softened. Transfer to a large bowl.

5. Add the beef, bread crumbs, milk, and thyme to the bowl. Season with salt and pepper and mix to combine.

6. In a small bowl, mix together the ketchup, brown sugar, and mustard.

7. Evenly divide the beef mixture between the cups of the prepared muffin tin.

8. Spoon the ketchup glaze onto each muffin.

9. Transfer the muffin tin to the oven, and bake for about 30 minutes, or until cooked through (internal temperature of 160°F). Remove from the oven.

MUSCLE-GAIN TIP: Increase the serving to 4 meat loaf muffins, and add a side of muscle-building quinoa.

PER SERVING (3 MEAT LOAVES): Calories: 323; Protein: 29g; Total carbohydrates: 38g; Fiber: 2g; Fat: 7g

MACROS: 35% Protein; 20% Fat; 45% Carbohydrates

Speedy Beef Stroganoff

PREP TIME: 15 minutes | COOK TIME: 25 minutes | Serves 4 | **MUSCLE GAIN**

Beef Stroganoff is classic comfort food, especially when spooned over egg noodles. The sauce is so luscious that sopping it up with bread may be desired. Try doubling the batch for leftovers. Purchase presliced beef to save time; it is usually labeled as stir-fry beef.

8 ounces whole wheat egg noodles

12 ounces sirloin steak, cut into thin strips

3 tablespoons all-purpose flour, divided

Sea salt

Freshly ground black pepper

2 teaspoons olive oil

2 cups low-sodium beef broth, divided

10 ounces white mushrooms, sliced

1 onion, chopped

2 teaspoons minced garlic

2 teaspoons Dijon mustard

1 teaspoon Worcestershire sauce

1 teaspoon chopped fresh thyme leaves

½ cup sour cream

1. Bring a large saucepan filled three-quarters full of water to a boil over high heat.

2. Add the noodles, and cook for about 12 minutes, or according to the package instructions. Remove from the heat. Drain.

3. While the noodles are cooking, put the steak in a plastic bag with 2 tablespoons of flour, the salt, and the pepper. Seal the bag, and shake gently to coat.

4. In a large skillet, heat the oil over medium-high heat.

5. Working in 2 batches, remove the steak from the bag, shake off the excess flour, and add the steak to the skillet. Cook for about 2½ minutes per batch, or until browned. Using a slotted spoon, transfer to a plate.

6. To make the sauce, to the skillet, add ¼ cup of broth, the mushrooms, onion, and garlic. Sauté for about 5 minutes, or until softened.

7. Whisk in the remaining 1 tablespoon of flour for 30 seconds.

8. Add the remaining 1¾ cups of broth, the mustard, the Worcestershire sauce, and the thyme. Bring to a boil, whisking.

9. Reduce the heat to medium-low. Simmer for about 5 minutes, or until the sauce has thickened.

10. Add the reserved steak with the juices on the plate and the sour cream. Stir to combine. Remove from the heat.

11. Serve the beef and sauce over the noodles.

FAT-LOSS TIP: Use Greek yogurt instead of sour cream to boost protein and reduce fat.

PER SERVING (¼ RECIPE): Calories: 462; Protein: 31g; Total carbohydrates: 54g; Fiber: 4g; Fat: 13g

MACROS: 27% Protein; 25% Fat; 48% Carbohydrates

Cheeseburger Bowls

PREP TIME: 15 minutes | COOK TIME: 10 minutes | Serves 3 | **MUSCLE GAIN**

Imagine all the flavors of a juicy cheeseburger in a bowl instead of on a bun. Although this dish is missing the bun, you can add a whole wheat roll as a side if so desired. Don't worry about the addition of lentils; they are mild tasting and do not detract from the balance of protein, vegetables, and cheese.

12 ounces extra-lean ground beef

1 teaspoon paprika

Sea salt

Freshly ground black pepper

2 (15-ounce) cans low-sodium lentils, drained and rinsed

6 cups shredded romaine lettuce

2 tomatoes, cut into chunks

½ cup shredded cheddar cheese

¼ cup chopped sweet pickles

¼ cup store-bought fat-free ranch or honey-mustard dressing

1. In a large skillet, sauté the beef over medium-high heat for about 6 minutes, or until cooked through. Remove from the heat. Drain any fat. Season with the paprika, salt, and pepper.

2. Fill 3 bowls halfway with the lentils.

3. Spoon the seasoned beef into the other half of each bowl.

4. Arrange the lettuce, tomatoes, cheese, and pickles in the bowls.

5. Drizzle with the dressing. Serve. Refrigerate the beef and lentils in 3 meal prep containers and the toppings in different containers for up to 3 days. Put together before serving.

FAT-LOSS TIP: Change this to a hamburger bowl by removing the cheese.

PER SERVING (⅓ RECIPE): Calories: 534; Protein: 49g; Total carbohydrates: 58g; Fiber: 20g; Fat: 14g

MACROS: 34% Protein; 23% Fat; 43% Carbohydrates

Sirloin and Bok Choy Stir-Fry

PREP TIME: 15 minutes | COOK TIME: 15 minutes | Serves 3 | **FAT LOSS**

Stir-frying is a culinary technique in which ingredients are cooked quickly over high heat. One of the tricks to ensure success is to cut the proteins and vegetables into uniform pieces.

¼ cup low-sodium beef broth

2 tablespoons low-sodium soy sauce

1 tablespoon maple syrup

1 tablespoon cornstarch

2 teaspoons sesame oil

1 teaspoon minced garlic

2 teaspoons olive oil

12 ounces sirloin steak, thinly sliced

2 cups water

1 cup whole wheat couscous

20 baby bok choy, quartered and thoroughly cleaned

2 red bell peppers, cored and sliced

2 scallions, both white and green parts, thinly sliced

1. In a small bowl, mix together the broth, soy sauce, maple syrup, cornstarch, sesame oil, and garlic and set aside.

2. In a large skillet, heat the olive oil over medium-high heat. Add the steak, and sauté for about 5 minutes, or until just cooked through. Using a slotted spoon, transfer to a plate.

3. While the steak is cooking, in a medium saucepan, bring the water to a boil over high heat.

4. Add the couscous. Remove from the heat. Cover the saucepan, and let stand for 10 minutes. Fluff with a fork.

5. Add the bok choy and bell peppers to the skillet. Sauté for about 5 minutes, or until tender-crisp.

6. Add the reserved sauce mixture and cook for about 5 minutes, or until thickened.

7. Add the steak back to the skillet, and toss to coat.

8. Serve the steak over the couscous, topped with the scallions.

MUSCLE-GAIN TIP: Add 6 ounces of sliced mushrooms along with the bok choy. Mushrooms are very high in vitamin D, which can play a role in muscle building.

PER SERVING (⅓ RECIPE): Calories: 402; Protein: 28g; Total carbohydrates: 51g; Fiber: 6g; Fat: 9g

MACROS: 28% Protein; 21% Fat; 51% Carbohydrates

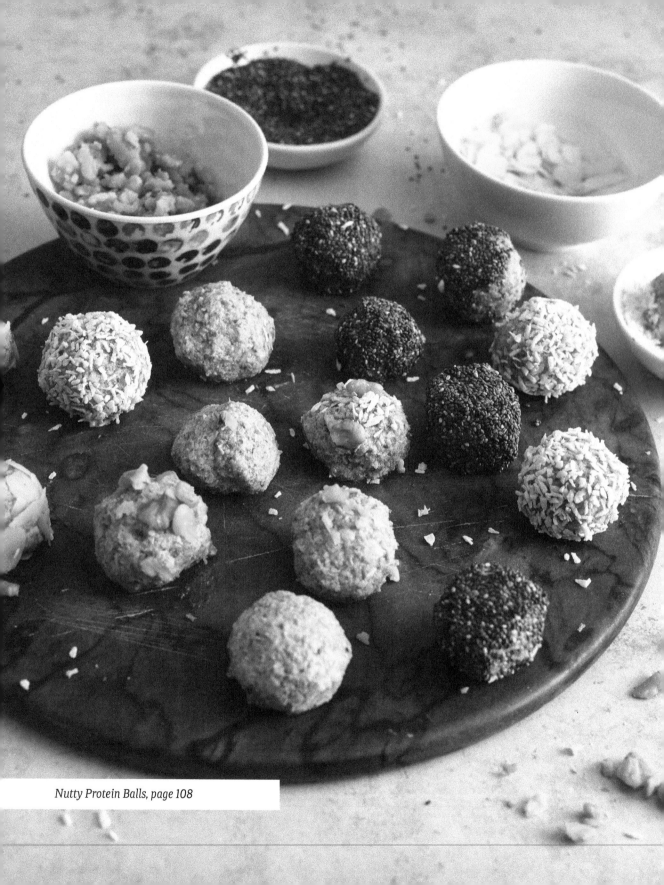

Nutty Protein Balls, page 108

CHAPTER 6

SNACKS AND DESSERTS

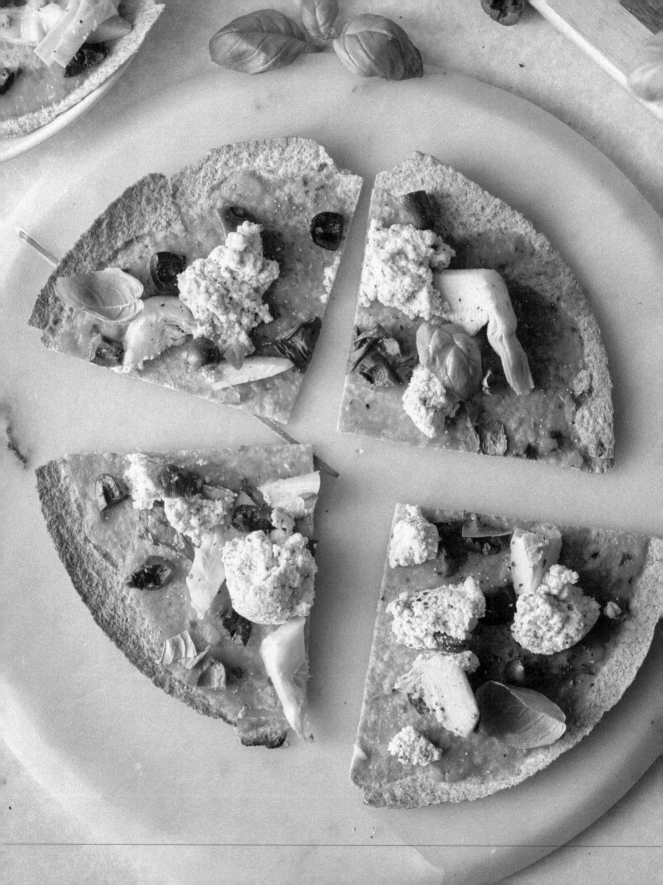

Mediterranean Tortilla Pizza

PREP TIME: 15 minutes | COOK TIME: 5 minutes | Serves 1 | **MUSCLE GAIN**

Prior to having thin-crust pizza in Malta in the late '80s, to me, pizza had always had puffy, bread-like crusts. Thin crust was an immediate favorite with the toppings front and center and the incredible crunch. Feel free to use a variety of toppings.

½ teaspoon extra-virgin olive oil

1 (10-inch) flour tortilla

2 tablespoons store-bought or homemade pizza sauce

¼ cup store-bought or homemade hummus

¼ cup canned artichoke hearts, drained and cut into eighths

¼ cup chopped black olives

Fresh basil, torn and whole leaves

Freshly ground black pepper

1. Set the oven to broil.

2. In a large, oven-safe skillet, heat the oil over medium-high heat.

3. Add the tortilla, and cook for about 1 minute, or until the underside is crispy.

4. Flip the tortilla over. Remove the skillet from the heat.

5. Spread the tortilla with the pizza sauce.

6. Add the hummus in teaspoons—do not spread it.

7. Top with the artichoke hearts and olives.

8. Transfer the skillet to the oven, and broil for about 2 minutes, or until the tortilla is very crispy. Remove from the oven.

9. Serve the pizza topped with fresh basil and seasoned with pepper.

FAT-LOSS TIP: Use an 8-inch tortilla, and scale down the toppings by one-quarter to cut the calories.

PER SERVING: Calories: 418; Protein: 12g; Total carbohydrates: 57g; Fiber: 10g; Fat: 15g
MACROS: 13% Protein; 32% Fat; 55% Carbohydrates

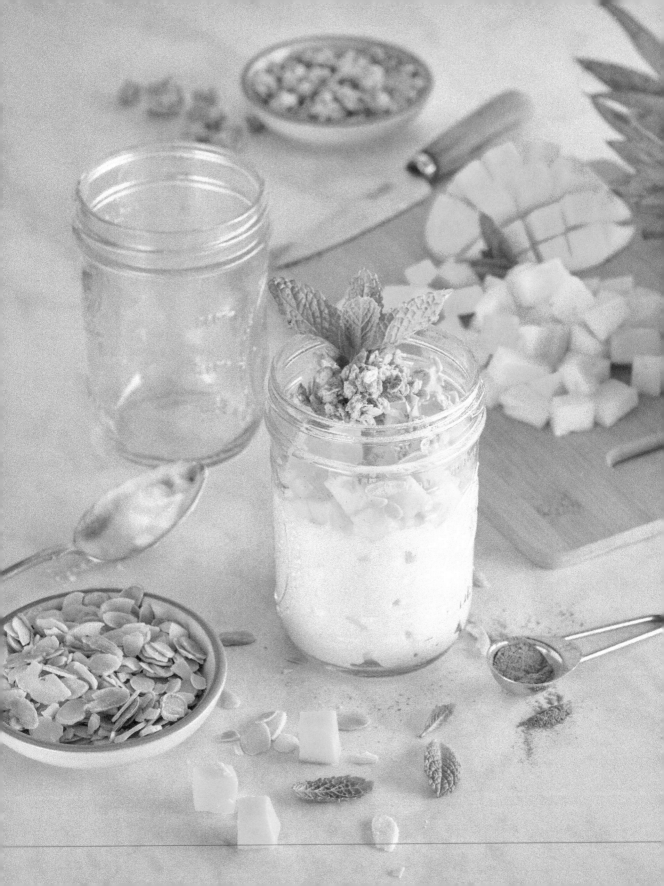

Tropical Cottage Cheese Parfait

PREP TIME: 15 minutes | COOK TIME: 25 minutes | Serves 4 | FAT LOSS

This fruity layered snack—or dessert—proves that a few simple ingredients can be delicious. And the addition of cottage cheese is excellent for fat loss and muscle gain. It is high protein, low calorie, and packed with vitamins and minerals. Not all of the granola will be used in this recipe, so save the rest to eat with a splash of milk.

¼ cup canola or melted coconut oil

¼ cup maple syrup

¼ teaspoon ground cinnamon

⅛ teaspoon ground nutmeg

⅛ teaspoon salt

2 cups rolled oats

¼ cup sliced almonds

¼ cup chopped walnuts

3 cups 2 percent cottage cheese

1 mango, peeled, pitted, and chopped

1 cup chopped pineapple (fresh or canned in 100 percent juice)

Mint sprigs, for topping (optional)

1. Preheat the oven to 300°F. Line a sheet pan with parchment paper.

2. To make the granola, in a medium bowl, mix together the oil, maple syrup, cinnamon, nutmeg, and salt until blended. Add the oats, almonds, and walnuts. Toss until everything is coated.

3. Spread the mixture out on the prepared sheet pan. Transfer the sheet pan to the oven, and bake, stirring halfway through, for about 25 minutes, or until the granola is golden. Remove from the oven. Let cool on the sheet pan, then transfer to an airtight container and store at room temperature for a week, or freeze for 1 month.

4. Evenly divide the cottage cheese between 4 canning jars or containers.

5. Evenly divide the mango and pineapple between the jars. Store in the refrigerator for up to 5 days.

6. Top with ¼ cup of the granola and mint (if using) just before serving.

MUSCLE-GAIN TIP: Switch out the 2 percent cottage cheese for full-fat.

PER SERVING (1 PARFAIT): Calories: 340; Protein: 23g; Total carbohydrates: 44g; Fiber: 5g; Fat: 10g

MACROS: 25% Protein; 25% Fat; 50% Carbohydrates

Nutty Protein Balls

PREP TIME: 20 minutes | Makes 12 to 14 balls | **MUSCLE GAIN**

These are like truffles but made with wholesome ingredients instead of chocolate and heaps of sugar. The protein powder adds flavor, so the choice of powder can affect the final taste profile. Try cookies and cream, pumpkin, or birthday cake for delicious variations.

1 cup almond butter

½ cup vanilla protein powder (vegan or unsweetened whey)

½ cup rolled oats

¼ cup unsweetened shredded coconut

2 tablespoons chia seeds

2 tablespoons honey

Shredded coconut, for topping (optional)

Sesame seeds, for topping (optional)

Chopped walnuts or pecans, for topping (optional)

Sliced almonds, for topping (optional)

1. In a large bowl, mix together the almond butter, protein powder, oats, coconut, chia seeds, and honey until combined.

2. Scoop up some batter, and press into a ball. If it crumbles apart, add water 1 teaspoon at a time until the batter stays together easily.

3. Using a tablespoon, scoop the batter, and roll into 1½-inch balls (12 to 14). Place in a container, and refrigerate for 1 hour or until firm. They can be refrigerated for up to 1 week, or frozen for up to 1 month.

FAT-LOSS TIP: These are quite filling, so even after cutting the portion in half, they are a satisfying snack.

PER SERVING (2 BALLS): Calories: 374; Protein: 19g; Total carbohydrates: 25g; Fiber: 7g; Fat: 49g

MACROS: 20% Protein; 53% Fat; 27% Carbohydrates

Dark Chocolate Fudge

PREP TIME: 10 minutes, plus 2 hours to freeze | Makes 36 pieces | **FAT LOSS**

Fudge is a decadent, creamy creation, ideal for treat meals, quick energy, or a mood lift. These squares are eaten straight from the freezer, and the texture is incredibly smooth. Try to use an extra chocolatey protein powder to boost the flavor.

½ cup milk or nondairy milk

⅓ cup peanut butter

3 scoops chocolate protein powder (vegan or whey)

2 tablespoons honey

1 teaspoon pure vanilla extract

1. Line a 6-inch square baking dish with parchment paper.

2. To make the batter, put the milk, peanut butter, protein powder, honey, and vanilla in a blender. Blend until very smooth.

3. Pour the batter into the baking dish, and smooth with a spatula. Freeze for about 2 hours, or until firm.

4. Cut the fudge into 36 (1-inch) pieces. Store in a sealed container in the freezer for up to 1 month.

MUSCLE-GAIN TIP: Add ¼ cup chopped cacao nibs for texture and epicatechin, a naturally occurring muscle-building chemical.

PER SERVING (4 PIECES): Calories: 113; Protein: 8g; Total carbohydrates: 10g; Fiber: 1g; Fat: 5g

MACROS: 30% Protein; 35% Fat; 35% Carbohydrates

Frozen Yogurt Bark

PREP TIME: 15 minutes, plus 2 hours to freeze | Serves 2 | FAT LOSS

Greek yogurt, maple syrup, and a hint of cinnamon freeze into cheesecake-like bark that breaks into jagged pieces. It can be taken right from the freezer to enjoy. Greek yogurt is an excellent source of protein, calcium, and probiotics, which are beneficial for both fat loss and muscle gain.

1 cup plain Greek yogurt

¼ cup chopped nuts, such as almonds, pecans, pistachios, or cashews

1 tablespoon maple syrup or honey

⅛ teaspoon ground cinnamon

Dried fruit, for topping (optional)

Mini chocolate chips, for topping (optional)

Seeds, for topping (optional)

1. Line a sheet pan with parchment paper.

2. In a medium bowl, mix together the yogurt, nuts, maple syrup, and cinnamon until well combined.

3. Using a spatula, spread the yogurt mixture out to a thickness of ½ to ¼ inch on the prepared sheet pan.

4. Top with dried fruit (if using), mini chocolate chips (if using), or seeds (if using). Freeze for about 2 hours, or until very firm.

5. Cut or break the bark into pieces; they do not have to be the same size. Store in a sealed container in the freezer for up to 1 month.

MUSCLE-GAIN TIP: Add ¼ cup pumpkin seeds; they are rich in muscle-building zinc.

PER SERVING: Calories: 182; Protein: 10g; Total carbohydrates: 19g; Fiber: 2g; Fat: 8g

MACROS: 23% Protein; 36% Fat; 41% Carbohydrates

Sesame-Oat Squares

PREP TIME: 10 minutes, plus 1 hour to chill | COOK TIME: 5 minutes
Makes 16 squares | **FAT LOSS**

These sesame treats don't snap in the same way that other sesame treats do, but the sesame taste is strong and delicious. Golden seeds are typically used, but any color will work.

¾ cup almond or peanut butter

¼ cup packed brown sugar

⅛ teaspoon ground cinnamon

1¼ cups rolled oats

¼ cup sesame seeds

1. Line an 8-inch square baking pan with parchment paper.

2. In a medium saucepan, combine the almond butter, brown sugar, and cinnamon. Cook, stirring, over medium heat for about 5 minutes, or until the mixture simmers and the sugar has dissolved. Remove from the heat.

3. Stir in the oats and sesame seeds.

4. Press the mixture into the prepared baking pan. Refrigerate for about 1 hour, or until firm.

5. Cut the mixture into 16 squares. Refrigerate in a sealed container for up to 1 week, or freeze for 1 month.

MUSCLE-GAIN TIP: Drizzle the bars with melted dark chocolate before refrigerating.

PER SERVING (1 SQUARE): Calories: 130; Protein: 5g; Total carbohydrates: 12g; Fiber: 3g; Fat: 8g

MACROS: 14% Protein; 48% Fat; 38% Carbohydrates

Chocolate Chip Cookie Dough Protein Balls

PREP TIME: 20 minutes | Makes 14 to 16 balls | **MUSCLE GAIN**

Cookie dough is trending as a snack. It's found as ice cream, smoothies, and bite-size treats. In fact, some of these snack products are made without eggs so they can be eaten right from the package. These protein balls have the same lovely vanilla flavor, chocolate morsels, and pleasing texture. And no eggs, either!

¾ cup almond butter

¼ cup honey

4 scoops vanilla protein powder (vegan or unsweetened whey)

2 teaspoons pure vanilla extract

½ cup oat flour

Sea salt

½ cup chocolate chips

1. In a large bowl, mix the almond butter, honey, protein powder, and vanilla until blended.

2. Stir in the oat flour and salt. Mix until a pressable dough forms.

3. Add the chocolate chips, and combine.

4. Scoop the dough out by heaping tablespoons, and roll into 14 to 16 balls. Put in a sealed container in the refrigerator to chill. Refrigerate for 1 hour or until firm. They can be refrigerated for up to 1 week, or frozen for 1 month.

FAT-LOSS TIP: Swap in 100 percent nuts peanut butter for the almond butter to cut the fat and calories.

PER SERVING (1 BALL): Calories: 176; Protein: 10g; Total carbohydrates: 18g; Fiber: 3g; Fat: 9g

MACROS: 20% Protein; 45% Fat; 35% Carbohydrates

Crispy Kale Chips

PREP TIME: 10 minutes | COOK TIME: 25 minutes | Serves 2 | **FAT LOSS**

These chips are low calorie with each portion containing almost 300 percent of the daily recommended amount of vitamin C. People deficient in this vitamin oxidize less fat during moderate exercise. The trick to very crispy chips is making sure the kale is completely dry before adding the oil.

4 cups kale, stemmed, thoroughly washed, and torn into 2-inch pieces

½ tablespoon olive oil

⅛ teaspoon sea salt

Ground cumin, for topping (optional)

Ground coriander, for topping (optional)

Paprika, for topping (optional)

Cayenne, for topping (optional)

Curry powder, for topping (optional)

Dried herbs, for topping (optional)

Garlic powder, for topping (optional)

Onion powder, for topping (optional)

1. Preheat the oven to 300°F. Line a sheet pan with parchment paper.

2. Using paper towels or a clean kitchen towel, dry the kale thoroughly, and transfer to a large bowl.

3. Toss the kale with the oil until each leaf is coated.

4. Spread the kale out in a single layer on the prepared sheet pan. Season with the salt.

5. Transfer the sheet pan to the oven, and bake, tossing halfway through, for about 25 minutes, or until the kale is dry and crispy. Remove from the oven. Transfer the kale to a cooling rack, and cool completely. Store at room temperature in a sealed container for up to 5 days.

6. When ready, serve the kale chips with cumin (if using), coriander (if using), paprika (if using), cayenne (if using), curry powder (if using), dried herbs (if using), garlic powder (if using), or onion powder (if using).

MUSCLE-GAIN TIP: It's okay to eat both portions here for 216 calories, so double up to increase kale's mineral contribution, like muscle-friendly magnesium and iron.

PER SERVING (½ RECIPE): Calories: 108; Protein: 6g; Total carbohydrates: 12g; Fiber: 1g; Fat: 4g

MACROS: 23% Protein; 32% Fat; 45% Carbohydrates

Avocado-Lime Deviled Eggs

PREP TIME: 20 minutes, plus at least 1 hour to chill | Serves 3 | **MUSCLE GAIN**

Deviled eggs are one of those snacks that magically disappear when they are available because they are delicious. Eggs are rich in high-quality protein, B vitamins, and the amino acid leucine, essential for muscle gain. The avocado adds healthy fats and a little fiber to round out these beauties.

6 large hard-boiled eggs, peeled

¼ cup mashed avocado

1 teaspoon freshly squeezed lime juice

Pinch cayenne

Sea salt

Freshly ground black pepper

1. Cut the eggs in half lengthwise. Carefully remove the yolks, and put in a medium bowl. Reserve the whites.

2. Add the avocado, lime juice, and cayenne to the yolks. Mix until very smooth and creamy. Season with salt and pepper.

3. Spoon the yolk mixture back into the egg white halves. Refrigerate for at least 1 hour before serving, then refrigerate for up to 2 days in a sealed container.

FAT-LOSS TIP: Make plain deviled eggs by omitting the avocado and using ¼ cup Greek yogurt instead. Top with a sprinkle of paprika.

PER SERVING (4 HALVES): Calories: 163; Protein: 13g; Total carbohydrates: 3g; Fiber: 1g; Fat: 11g

MACROS: 37% Protein; 57% Fat; 6% Carbohydrates

Roasted Chickpeas

PREP TIME: 10 minutes | COOK TIME: 30 minutes | Serves 4 | FAT LOSS

Chickpeas are incredible roasted; they become satisfyingly crunchy, with a nutty flavor reminiscent of sesame seeds. This recipe is merely the base; it's delicious as is, but feel free to add any desired seasoning. Try spice blends such as ras el hanout or garam masala.

2 (15-ounce) cans no-salt-added chickpeas, drained and rinsed

1 tablespoon olive oil

1 teaspoon ground cumin, for topping (optional)

1 teaspoon paprika, for topping (optional)

1 teaspoon Italian seasoning, for topping (optional)

1 teaspoon ground coriander, for topping (optional)

1 teaspoon curry powder, for topping (optional)

Sea salt

1. Preheat the oven to 375°F. Line a sheet pan with parchment paper.

2. Using paper towels or a clean kitchen towel, dry the chickpeas thoroughly.

3. In a medium bowl, toss together the chickpeas and oil until well coated.

4. Add the cumin (if using), paprika (if using), Italian seasoning (if using), coriander (if using), or curry powder (if using).

5. Spread the chickpeas out evenly on the prepared sheet pan.

6. Transfer the sheet pan to the oven, and bake, stirring halfway through, for about 30 minutes, or until the chickpeas are crisp and golden. Remove from the oven. Season lightly with salt. Let cool completely on the sheet pan. Store in a sealed container at room temperature for up to 5 days.

MUSCLE-GAIN TIP: Increase the portion for extra calories; the macros are excellent for muscle gain and fat loss.

PER SERVING (¼ RECIPE): Calories: 232; Protein: 11g; Total carbohydrates: 34g; Fiber: 9g; Fat: 7g

MACROS: 19% Protein; 24% Fat; 57% Carbohydrates

Cheesy Crab Dip

PREP TIME: 10 minutes | COOK TIME: 15 minutes | Serves 3 | **MUSCLE GAIN**

Sometimes a cheesy, decadent dip with crunchy dippers is needed to satisfy snack cravings, so here is a perfect choice. Crab isn't just high in protein; it is also an excellent source of fatty acids, calcium, and iron. Look for quality frozen or canned crab for the best results, and check the label to ensure there is no added sodium.

6 ounces cream cheese, at room temperature

½ cup grated Parmesan cheese

⅓ cup sour cream

Juice of 1 lime

½ teaspoon minced garlic

Pinch red pepper flakes

1 (6-ounce) can crabmeat, drained

Sea salt

Freshly ground black pepper

¼ cup shredded cheddar cheese

Cut vegetables, naan, or tortilla crisps, for dipping

1. Preheat the oven to 400° F.

2. In a medium bowl, stir together the cream cheese, Parmesan cheese, sour cream, lime juice, garlic, and red pepper flakes.

3. Add the crab. Season with salt and pepper. Transfer to an oven-safe 3-cup bowl.

4. Top with the cheddar cheese.

5. Transfer the bowl to the oven, and bake for about 15 minutes, or until the dip is golden and bubbling. Remove from the oven. Serve hot with the cut vegetables, naan, or tortilla crisps. Refrigerate any leftovers in an airtight container for up to 3 days.

FAT-LOSS TIP: Swap in low-fat cream cheese, low-fat sour cream, and low-fat cheddar.

PER SERVING: Calories: 311; Protein: 20g; Total carbohydrates: 7g; Fiber: 0g; Fat: 23g

MACROS: 25% Protein; 64% Fat; 11% Carbohydrates

Chocolate-Chili Pudding

PREP TIME: 15 minutes, plus 3 hours to chill | COOK TIME: 10 minutes | Serves 4
FAT LOSS

Chocolate and chili are a traditional pairing; the chili seems to heighten the richness of the chocolate. Chili contains an active compound called capsaicin that revs the metabolism to support weight loss. Feel free to add a couple of pinches of cayenne to boost the heat.

3 cups nondairy or regular milk

1 cup light coconut milk

2 teaspoons pure vanilla extract

½ cup unsweetened cocoa powder

⅓ cup sugar

¼ cup arrowroot flour

⅛ teaspoon chili powder

Sea salt

1. In a medium saucepan, combine the milk, coconut milk, and vanilla. Heat over medium heat until just simmering. Remove from the heat.

2. In a small bowl, whisk together the cocoa powder, sugar, flour, chili powder, and salt until no lumps remain.

3. Whisk the dry mixture into the wet mixture until well blended. Bring to a simmer, whisking constantly, for about 3 minutes, or until thickened. Remove from the heat. Pour into a bowl, and cover with plastic wrap so the wrap presses on the top. Refrigerate for about 3 hours, or until completely cooled. Serve.

MUSCLE-GAIN TIP: Add sliced almonds to the pudding to add muscle-building protein and magnesium.

PER SERVING (¼ RECIPE): Calories: 298; Protein: 10g; Total carbohydrates: 40g; Fiber: 5g; Fat: 12g

MACROS: 13% Protein; 37% Fat; 50% Carbohydrates

Peanut Butter–Banana Mousse

PREP TIME: 10 minutes | Serves 4 | **MUSCLE GAIN**

This recipe uses peanut flour—which can be found in the organic section of most grocery stores—to create a luscious, decadent dessert. This ingredient adds an intense peanut flavor without as much fat as the popular butter, and the flour fluffs up the texture when added to the other ingredients.

1 (14-ounce) block extra-firm tofu, drained and pressed (see page 43)

2 cups peanut flour

1½ cups milk or nondairy milk

2 tablespoons maple syrup

1 tablespoon pure vanilla extract

Sea salt

1 banana, peeled and thinly sliced

1. Put the tofu, peanut flour, milk, maple syrup, vanilla, and salt in a blender. Blend until very smooth and fluffy, scraping down the sides with a spatula.

2. Serve the mousse topped with the banana. Refrigerate any leftovers in a sealed container for up to 4 days.

FAT-LOSS TIP: Use skim milk instead of whole milk to reduce the fat content.

PER SERVING (¼ RECIPE): Calories: 349; Protein: 24g; Total carbohydrates: 34g; Fiber: 6g; Fat: 13g

MACROS: 28% Protein; 32% Fat; 40% Carbohydrates

Maple-Walnut Quinoa Pudding

PREP TIME: 5 minutes | COOK TIME: 25 minutes | Serves 4 | FAT LOSS

Any grain can be made into a creamy, comforting pudding; quinoa takes the place of the usual rice in this version. Maple-walnut is a favorite ice cream in our home, so this recipe was created with this in mind. Although not exactly ice cream, it is delicious!

2 cups milk or unsweetened nondairy milk

1 cup quinoa, rinsed

⅓ cup maple syrup

½ teaspoon ground cinnamon

Pinch ground cloves

Sea salt

½ cup chopped walnuts

1. In a large saucepan, stir together the milk, quinoa, maple syrup, cinnamon, cloves, and salt over medium heat. Bring to a simmer, stirring occasionally.

2. Reduce the heat to low. Simmer for about 20 minutes, or until the liquid has been absorbed by the quinoa. Remove from the heat.

3. Stir in the walnuts. Serve, or let cool completely and store in the refrigerator for up to 1 week. Reheat with a little extra milk.

MUSCLE-GAIN TIP: Add ¼ cup hemp hearts to boost protein by 3 grams per portion.

PER SERVING (¼ RECIPE): Calories: 381; Protein: 13g; Total carbohydrates: 53g; Fiber: 4g; Fat: 14g

MACROS: 15% Protein; 32% Fat; 53% Carbohydrates

WORKOUT ROUTINES

This section offers workout routines organized by fat loss and muscle gain, with numerous illustrations for guidance. Each routine provides cardio, HIIT, and strength-training routines. Although the workout routines themselves need not change based on which category someone sits in, the relative frequency and priority of each may change.

An individual looking primarily for fat loss, for example, can regularly engage in resistance training but may opt instead to focus more on HIIT or cardio because resistance training may not be as important to their individual goals as it is to someone trying to add muscle.

Fat Loss

CARDIO

Cardiovascular activity has a number of physical and mental health benefits and can be an effective complement to proper nutrition when it comes to supporting a primary goal of fat loss. The type of cardio will depend on preferences and capabilities and may range across modalities such as running, swimming, biking, rowing, or the elliptical.

Most sports tend to fall between the "Cardio" and "HIIT" range, and so those who engage in any weekly sporting activity could count that in this category as well. What we are looking for from cardiovascular workouts is a moderate intensity and moderate duration.

Aim for a 30- to 40-minute commitment to the activity of choice with an eye on performance. Performance can be measured by how much distance is being covered in X amount of time on a weekly basis and working to gradually increase distance, speed, or both over time.

Cardio may be performed 1 to 3 times weekly, depending on preference.

HIIT

Unlike the cardio described previously, HIIT is more of a high-intensity and low- to moderate-duration type of activity that involves working near your limits in a manner that is spaced out by rest intervals and for an overall duration that is generally less than traditional cardio workouts.

HIIT workouts can be carried out in a variety of ways and expend more energy in less time, so the time commitment is 20 to 30 minutes to spend the same amount of energy as the steady-state cardio depicted previously.

Routine Option #1: Run/Walk/Sprint Intervals

For those who struggle with steady-state cardiovascular training, interval sprints are probably the next-best alternative. Note that this style of training can also be applied to other forms of cardio as well. The goal here is to alternate between bouts of walking (low intensity), jogging (moderate intensity), and sprinting (high intensity) for a period of at least 20 minutes, broken up into equal intervals of 15 to 20 seconds or a duration of your preference. Beginners may opt to choose longer walk/jog intervals and shorter sprint intervals.

Routine Option #2: Jump Rope Intervals

Jumping rope represents a very effective and straightforward HIIT style workout. Twenty seconds of intense jump rope with 10 seconds rest, repeated over a 20-minute duration, will do the trick.

STRENGTH TRAINING

Strength training remains an important and relevant consideration in any fitness routine, even when adding muscle is not the goal. Strength training can be incorporated at a lower frequency (for example, once per week rotating through each workout on a weekly basis), depending on personal preference.

The strength workouts are presented in three categories: push muscles, pull muscles, and legs. Each workout includes 3 primary exercises that are to be completed for a minimum of 3 sets and at 8 to 12 repetitions, depending on the nature of the exercise. Note that activities involving weights should be completed with 3 to 5 sets for 8 to 12 reps. For activities involving body weight, complete 3 to 5 sets of max reps.

Routine Option #1: Push Muscles

- Bench presses (barbell/dumbbell) or shoulder presses (barbell/dumbbell) (page 125)

- Overhead press (page 125)

- Dips or push-ups (easier on shoulder press days) (page 126)

- Lying tricep extensions (page 126)

Routine Option #2: Pull Muscles

- Pull-ups (page 127)

- Inverted rows (body weight or one-arm) (page 127)

- Hammer curls (page 128)

Routine Option #3: Legs

- Back squat (page 129)

- Stiff-leg dead lift (page 129)

Tracking and recording progress around the advancement to higher weights or higher rep counts is a process known as "progressive overload" and will help support muscle-gain goals.

Muscle Gain

Whether the primary goal is significant muscle gain or modest muscle gain paired with some level of fat loss, resistance training should be the focal point of the routine. Although the relative frequency of resistance training to cardiovascular and HIIT style training is ultimately a personal choice, a minimum of three resistance workouts per week is the expectation. More experienced individuals may opt for four to six resistance workouts a week, but this may not be advisable for beginners who will require sufficient time to recover and adapt.

Those interested in maintaining cardiovascular fitness may want to incorporate either HIIT, cardio, or some form of sports at least once a week or even multiple times a week. Mobility-type workouts like yoga or stretching may also have a role to play to prevent injuries and maintain mobility while gaining muscle.

CARDIO

Cardiovascular activity has a number of physical and mental health benefits, and maintaining some level of cardiovascular fitness is beneficial even in the presence of a muscle-gain goal. The type of cardio will depend on personal preferences and may range across modalities such as running, swimming, biking, rowing, or the elliptical.

Most sports tend to fall between the "Cardio" and "HIIT" range, and so those who engage in any weekly sporting activity could count that in this category as well. The goal with cardiovascular endeavors is a moderate intensity and moderate duration. Aim for 30 to 40 minutes of commitment to the activity of choice with an eye on performance, meaning how much distance is being covered in X amount of time on a weekly basis. Can you gradually increase it? Try for at least one or two cardio or HIIT workouts per week, depending on what resistance training frequency allows.

HIIT

Here are two high-intensity routines for muscle gain.

Routine Option #1: Run/Walk/Sprint Intervals

For those who struggle to get excited for steady-state cardiovascular training, interval sprints probably represent the next-best alternative. Note that this style of training can also be applied to other forms of cardio as well. The goal is to alternate between bouts of walking (low intensity), jogging (moderate intensity), and sprinting (high intensity) for a period of at least 20 minutes.

Routine Option #2: Jump Rope Intervals

Jumping rope represents a very effective and straightforward HIIT-style workout. Twenty seconds of intense jump rope with 10 seconds rest repeated over a 20-minute duration can do the trick.

STRENGTH TRAINING

Strength training is the foundational component of any training regimen focused on gaining muscle and requires a minimum of three workouts weekly.

The strength workouts are presented in three categories: push muscles, pull muscles, and legs. Each workout includes 3 primary exercises to be completed for a minimum of 3 sets and at 8 to 12 repetitions, depending on the nature of the exercise. Note that activities involving weights should be completed with 3 to 5 sets for 8 to 12 reps. For activities involving body weight, complete 3 to 5 sets of max reps.

Routine Option #1: Push Muscles

- Bench presses (barbell/dumbbell) or shoulder presses (barbell/dumbbell) (page 125)

- Overhead press (page 125)

- Dips or push-ups (easier on shoulder press days) (page 126)

- Lying tricep extensions (page 126)

Routine Option #2: Pull Muscles

- Pull-ups (page 127)

- Inverted rows (body weight or one-arm) (page 127)

- Hammer curls (page 128)

Routine Option #3: Legs

- Back squat (page 129)

- Stiff-leg dead lift (page 129)

Exercise Examples

Bench Press (barbell or dumbbell)

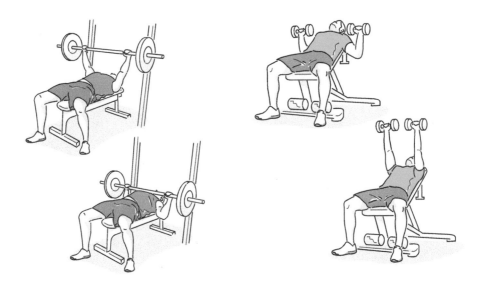

Overhead Press

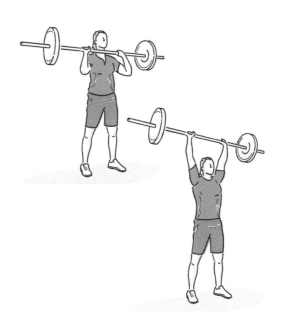

PUSH DAY (cont.)

Push-Ups/Dips

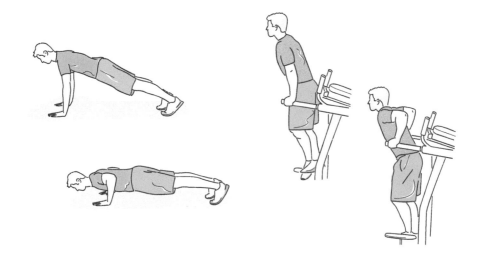

Lying Tricep Extension

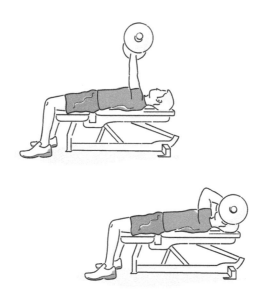

PULL DAY

Pull-Up

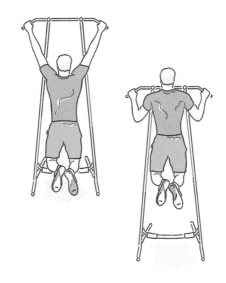

Inverted Rows

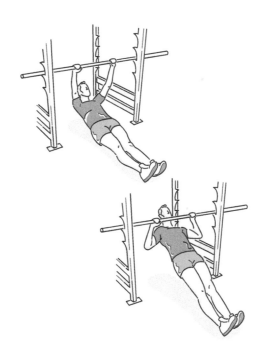

PULL DAY (cont.)

Hammer Curl

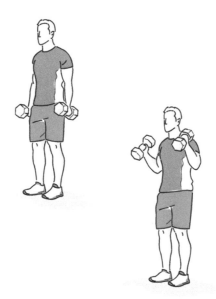

LEG DAY

Back Squat

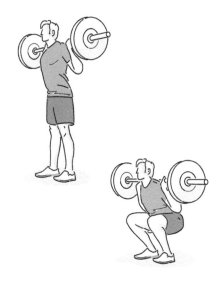

Stiff-Leg Deadlift (barbell or dumbbell)

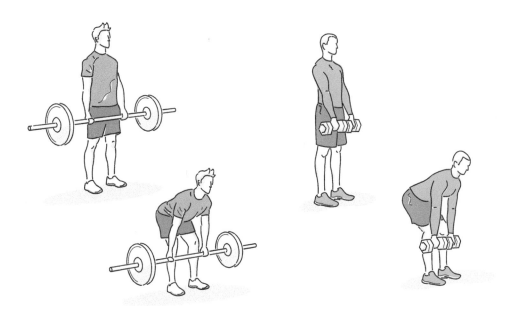

MEASUREMENT CONVERSIONS

VOLUME EQUIVALENTS	U.S. STANDARD	U.S. STANDARD (OUNCES)	METRIC (APPROXIMATE)
LIQUID	2 tablespoons	1 fl. oz.	30 mL
	¼ cup	2 fl. oz.	60 mL
	½ cup	4 fl. oz.	120 mL
	1 cup	8 fl. oz.	240 mL
	1½ cups	12 fl. oz.	355 mL
	2 cups or 1 pint	16 fl. oz.	475 mL
	4 cups or 1 quart	32 fl. oz.	1 L
	1 gallon	128 fl. oz.	4 L
DRY	⅛ teaspoon	—	0.5 mL
	¼ teaspoon	—	1 mL
	½ teaspoon	—	2 mL
	¾ teaspoon	—	4 mL
	1 teaspoon	—	5 mL
	1 tablespoon	—	15 mL
	¼ cup	—	59 mL
	⅓ cup	—	79 mL
	½ cup	—	118 mL
	⅔ cup	—	156 mL
	¾ cup	—	177 mL
	1 cup	—	235 mL
	2 cups or 1 pint	—	475 mL
	3 cups	—	700 mL
	4 cups or 1 quart	—	1 L
	½ gallon	—	2 L
	1 gallon	—	4 L

OVEN TEMPERATURES

FAHRENHEIT	CELSIUS (APPROXIMATE)
250°F	120°C
300°F	150°C
325°F	165°C
350°F	180°C
375°F	190°C
400°F	200°C
425°F	220°C
450°F	230°C

WEIGHT EQUIVALENTS

U.S. STANDARD	METRIC (APPROXIMATE)
½ ounce	15 g
1 ounce	30 g
2 ounces	60 g
4 ounces	115 g
8 ounces	225 g
12 ounces	340 g
16 ounces or 1 pound	455 g

REFERENCES

Chin, Edwin C., Angus P. Yu, Christopher W. Lai, Daniel Y. Fong, Derwin K. Chan, Stephen H. Wong, Fenghua Sun, Heidi H. Ngai, Patrick S. H. Yung, and Parco M. Siu. "Low-Frequency HIIT Improves Body Composition and Aerobic Capacity in Overweight Men." *Medicine & Science in Sports & Exercise* 52, no. 1 (January 2020): 56–66. doi.org/10.1249/ MSS.0000000000002097.

Kreider, Richard B., Douglas S. Kalman, Jose Antonio, Tim N. Ziegenfuss, Robert Wildman, Rick Collins, Darren G. Candow, Susan M. Kleiner, Anthony L. Almada, and Hector L. Lopez. "International Society of Sports Nutrition Position Stand: Safety and Efficacy of Creatine Supplementation in Exercise, Sport, and Medicine." *Journal of the International Society of Sports Nutrition* 14, no. 18 (June 2017). doi.org/10.1186/s12970-017-0173-z.

Schoenfeld, Brad Jon, and Alan Albert Aragon. "How Much Protein Can the Body Use in a Single Meal for Muscle-Building? Implications for Daily Protein Distribution." *Journal of the International Society of Sports Nutrition* 15, 10 (February 2018). doi.org/10.1186 /s12970-018-0215-1.

Swift, Damon L., Neil M. Johannsen, Carl J. Lavie, Conrad P. Earnest, and Timothy S. Church. "The Role of Exercise and Physical Activity in Weight Loss and Maintenance." *Progress in Cardiovascular Diseases* 56, no. 4 (January/February 2014): 441–7. doi.org/10.1016/j .pcad.2013.09.012.

Whittaker, Joseph, and Kexin Wu. "Low-Fat Diets and Testosterone in Men: Systematic Review and Meta-Analysis of Intervention Studies." *Journal of Steroid Biochemistry and Molecular Biology* 210 (June 2021). doi.org/10.1016/j.jsbmb.2021.105878.

Zhang, Haifeng, Tom K. Tong, Weifeng Qiu, Xu Zhang, Shi Zhou, Yang Liu, and Yuxiu He. "Comparable Effects of High-Intensity Interval Training and Prolonged Continuous Exercise Training on Abdominal Visceral Fat Reduction in Obese Young Women." *Journal of Diabetes Research* 2017 (January 2017). doi.org/10.1155/2017/5071740.

INDEX

About the Author

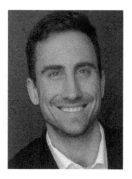 **Andy De Santis, RD, MPH,** is a private practice dietitian and published author from Toronto. He graduated in 2014 from the University of Toronto School of Public Health with a master's degree and has gone on to write nine books and hundreds of blog posts while working with individuals to tailor a nutrition strategy to fit their personal goals. He brings a wealth of nutrition science knowledge and tailored nutrition solutions to this book in order to eliminate any guesswork so that readers can clearly pursue their fitness goals.

CPSIA information can be obtained
at www.ICGtesting.com
Printed in the USA
JSHW021708130222
22794JS00003B/4